DID YOU KNOW ...

... that babies born to women with diabetes have a 97–98% survival rate—nearly as high as that of babies whose mothers don't have diabetes?

... that you don't nece... alto-gether, if you have dia...

... that there *are* succe... ...n who become impotent from dia...

GETTING THE FACTS ABOUT DIABETES IS THE FIRST STEP TOWARD FEELING GOOD AND STAY-ING HEALTHY. UP-TO-DATE, RELIABLE INFOR-MATION; REASSURING ANSWERS; AND STRAIGHT TALK ABOUT SELF-CARE CAN ALL BE YOURS WITH ...

LIVING WITH DIABETES

ARLAN L. ROSENBLOOM, M.D., is a professor in the Col-lege of Medicine at the University of Florida in Gainesville, and founding director of the University of Florida Diabetes Center. He has served on numerous national advisory boards, including the Board of the American Diabetes Association and the National Diabetes Advisory at the National Institute of Health.
DIANA TONNESSEN has written several books on health and medicine. A former managing editor at *Health* magazine, she lives in Gainesville, Florida.

LIVING WITH Diabetes

*A Comprehensive Guide to
Understanding and Controlling Diabetes
While Enjoying Your Life*

ARLAN L. ROSENBLOOM, M.D., AND DIANA TONNESSEN

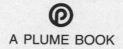
A PLUME BOOK

PLUME
Published by the Penguin Group
Penguin Books USA Inc., 375 Hudson Street,
New York, New York 10014, U.S.A.
Penguin Books Ltd, 27 Wrights Lane, London W8 5TZ, England
Penguin Books Australia Ltd, Ringwood, Victoria, Australia
Penguin Books Canada Ltd, 10 Alcorn Avenue,
Toronto, Ontario, Canada M4V 3B2
Penguin Books (N.Z.) Ltd, 182–190 Wairau Road, Auckland 10, New Zealand

Penguin Books Ltd, Registered Offices: Harmondsworth, Middlesex, England

First published by Plume, an imprint of Dutton Signet,
a division of Penguin Books USA Inc.

First Printing, December, 1993
10 9 8 7 6 5 4

High-Fiber Foods table beginning on page 29 excerpted with permission from Anderson, James W., *Plant Fiber in Foods*. Lexington, Kentucky, HCF Nutrition Research Foundation., Inc., 1990. Copyright 1990 by James W. Anderson, M.D.

The Exchange Values for Alcoholic Beverages on page 43 reprinted with permission from the *Physician's Guide to Insulin-Dependent (Type I) Diabetes.* Copyright 1988 American Diabetes Association, Inc.

Guidelines for Eating Out list beginning on page 52 reprinted with permission from Davidson, Meyer B., *Diabetes Mellitus: Diagnosis and Treatment* (third edition), Churchill Livingstone, New York, 1991.

Medications that May Cause Drug Interactions with Oral Hypoglycemic Agents list beginning on page 72 reprinted with permission from the *Physician's Guide to Non-Insulin-Dependent (Type II) Diabetes.* Copyright 1989 American Diabetes Association, Inc.

 REGISTERED TRADEMARK—MARCA REGISTRADA

LIBRARY OF CONGRESS CATALOGING IN PUBLICATION DATA:
Rosenbloom, Arlan L.
    Living with diabetes : a comprehensive guide to understanding and controlling diabetes while enjoying your life / Arlan L. Rosenbloom and Diana Tonnessen.
    p. cm.
    ISBN 0-452-27093-6
    1. Diabetes—Popular works. I. Tonnessen, Diana. II. Title.
RC660.4.R68—1993
362.1′96462—dc20   93–22801
                                                                    CIP

Printed in the United States of America
Designed by Eve L. Kirch

ACKNOWLEDGMENTS

Special thanks to

Donna Greenwood, M.Ed., R.D.
Martha McCallum, B.S.N., R.N., C.D.E.
Betsey Neis
Peggy Polopolus
Bonnie Prescott
Rita Revak-Lutz, M.S.N., A.R.N.P., C.D.E.

Contents

Contents

CHAPTER 1

Myths and Misconceptions

"It can't be diabetes," you exclaim as your physician reviews the results of your diagnostic tests. "There must be some mistake!" Whether or not you have one or more of the classic symptoms of diabetes—frequent urination, excessive thirst, sudden weight loss, constant fatigue—finding out you have diabetes can be quite a shock. After all, diabetes is not like a cold or the flu; it doesn't go away—even when you get the best medical care possible.

If you have symptoms, you can take some comfort in knowing that you'll feel much better once your diabetes has been diagnosed and treated. But what about all those horror stories you've heard about the disease? Will you have to take insulin shots? Will you have to give up treats for the rest of your life? Isn't it too risky for people with diabetes to have children? And what about blindness, amputations, heart disease, and other serious long-term complications? Is there any chance of leading a normal, productive life?

Because diabetes is fairly common (some 6 million Americans have been diagnosed), much of what you have heard about the disease has probably come from family or friends, the popular press, or movies and television. But as the message filters down, it often gets misinterpreted, oversimplified, or misstated. So many of your impressions about diabetes may not be accurate—or up to date with the current research.

Misinformation about diabetes raises a lot of needless fear and confusion. Too often, those fears stand in the way of getting the necessary treatment—particularly if you don't *feel* sick (at least not right now). *But diabetes is most dangerous when it is left untreated.* Whether or not you have symptoms, you have the best chance of leading a long, productive, and healthy life when your diabetes is kept under control. To help ease your fears, let's look at some of the misconceptions many people have about the disease.

MYTH: All people with diabetes must take insulin shots.

FACT: Most people with diabetes *don't* have to take insulin shots. As you may already be aware, there are two major forms of diabetes: Type I, or insulin-dependent diabetes, and Type II, or non-insulin-dependent diabetes. People with Type I diabetes produce little or no *insulin*, a hormone secreted from the pancreas gland behind the stomach. Insulin helps your body's tissues store and use the sugars *(glucose)*, protein, and fats circulating in your bloodstream after you eat a meal. Without insulin, people with Type I diabetes can't process or use the food they eat for energy. In effect, their bodies starve, even though they eat plenty of food. These people *must* take insulin shots to survive; hence the name insulin-dependent diabetes, the term we will use throughout this book.

Only about 10 percent of all people with diabetes have insulin-dependent diabetes. Most people have Type II diabetes. These people produce insulin, but often in inadequate amounts. Moreover, the insulin that the body does produce isn't used efficiently, resulting in what's known as *insulin resistance*. And while some people with Type II diabetes may have to take insulin to lower dangerously elevated blood sugar levels, insulin shots aren't necessary for survival; hence the name non-insulin-dependent diabetes.

The good news about non-insulin-dependent diabetes is that most people can control it with lifestyle changes alone. In fact, if you are overweight, you may find that simply losing weight is all you need to do to keep your diabetes in check.

MYTH: Adults don't get "juvenile" diabetes and children don't get "adult-onset" diabetes.

FACT: In the past, insulin-dependent diabetes was called juvenile-onset diabetes because most people who develop diabetes before age twenty-five have this form of the disease. But you can develop insulin-dependent diabetes at any age.

Likewise, non-insulin-dependent diabetes was once referred to as adult-onset diabetes because most people who develop this form of diabetes are over forty. But older children, adolescents, and young adults can develop non-insulin-dependent diabetes as well.

MYTH: Diabetes is caused by eating too many sweets.

FACT: No one knows exactly what causes diabetes. We do know that eating a lot of sugar does not in itself cause diabetes. But eating too many sugar- and fat-laden sweets *can* cause you to gain weight. And being overweight is one of the major risk factors for non-insulin-dependent diabetes.

Scientists now know that insulin-dependent diabetes is an *autoimmune disease*, in which the body's immune defense system for some reason turns on its own tissues. In people with insulin-dependent diabetes, antibodies formed by the immune system attack and destroy the insulin-producing beta cells of the pancreas. *Why* this occurs in some people is still a mystery, but it has nothing to do with having an overactive sweet tooth.

Your genes play a role in the development of diabetes, too. Scientists have found that a cluster of genes that governs the regulation of the body's immune defense system is associated with a genetic risk for insulin-dependent diabetes. And while the same genes aren't associated with non-insulin-dependent diabetes, this form of diabetes has a hereditary component as well. Studies involving identical twins, who share the same genes, show that if one twin develops non-insulin-dependent diabetes, there is a 90 to 100 percent chance that the other twin will, too.

MYTH: People with diabetes shouldn't have children because they might pass it on to their offspring.

FACT: The majority of people with insulin-dependent diabetes *do not* have a family history of the disease. Fewer than 5 percent of all children whose parents have insulin-dependent diabetes go on to develop the disease themselves. For non-insulin-dependent diabetes the risk for relatives is considerably higher. Remember, though, that what people inherit is a genetic predisposition to diabetes that can be triggered by lifestyle habits, such as diet and exercise—*not* the disease itself.

Some of the most promising new research in diabetes now suggests that both types of diabetes can be prevented in high-risk people (more on this later). Even if your children do go on to develop diabetes, it's not such a terrible fate—as you will soon see. For the most part, people with diabetes can do anything other people can do. Keep in mind, too, that research is leading to improved screening tests and new treatments, and may one day result in a cure—perhaps in your children's lifetime. When you think about it, if you want to have children, the pain of not having them may be far more devastating than the possibility of passing on a legacy of diabetes.

MYTH: Women with diabetes should not have children. It's too dangerous.

FACT: If you saw the movie *Steel Magnolias*, in which actress Julia Roberts plays a woman with insulin-dependent diabetes whose decision to have a baby costs her life, you probably got the impression that having a family is just too risky for women with diabetes. Pregnancy is risky for *any* woman, and while certain pregnancy-related health risks are somewhat greater for women with diabetes, you can reduce the risks to you and your baby by maintaining good control of your blood sugar. In fact, if you diligently control your diabetes before you conceive and throughout your pregnancy, *your chances of having a healthy baby are about the same as those of a woman who doesn't have diabetes.* (You'll learn the ways in which you can reduce your risk during pregnancy, including which specialist you should see, in Chapter 9.)

MYTH: People with diabetes can't eat sweets.

FACT: People with diabetes should avoid excess sweets largely because these foods are fattening and cause tooth decay. But there's no scientific reason that you can't occasionally and judiciously indulge.

MYTH: Nothing can be done to prevent the long-term complications of diabetes, such as heart disease, kidney problems, loss of eyesight, or nerve damage, so there's no point in knocking yourself out to control your diabetes.

FACT: Medical scientists have recognized that the long-term complications of diabetes such as kidney damage, eye changes that can threaten vision, and nerve damage, were more likely to occur in people with the least well-controlled blood sugar levels. But they also recognized that many people with the best control possible by the means available until just a few years ago also developed these complications. The question was whether it was possible to achieve a degree of control that could prevent or greatly delay these problems using newer methods of giving insulin and monitoring control. Numerous small studies suggested that good control of blood sugar levels might delay the onset and slow the progression of the complications of the disease. Now, a landmark ten-year study, the Diabetes Control and Complications Trial, sponsored by the National Institute of Diabetes and Digestive and Kidney Disease, has confirmed the results of these smaller studies and has shown that diligent control of diabetes can reduce the incidence and severity of complications.

The study, involving 1,441 people with insulin-dependent diabetes, compared the effects of two forms of therapy: conventional and intensive. Those receiving conventional care—the kind currently prescribed for most people with insulin-dependent diabetes—took one or two insulin injections per day, tested their blood sugar once a day, and followed the standard advice about nutrition and exercise. Those receiving intensive therapy took three to five insulin injections per day or used an insulin pump, and tested their blood four to seven times a day with the goal of keeping their blood sugar as close to normal as possible. They also maintained close contact with their diabetes care team, who called them on the phone one or more times a week.

The researchers reported an approximately 60 percent reduction in risk for the development and progression of eye disease, kidney damage, and nerve damage in the group of people who maintained tight control of their blood sugar levels, compared to the group receiving standard care. According to this study, the more normal your blood glucose level is, the lower is your risk of developing complications. The researchers believe the same tight control of blood sugar levels will help prevent complications in people with non-insulin-dependent diabetes, as well.

You should be aware, however, that tight control carries its own risks: the people receiving intensive care are three times as likely to pass out from low blood sugar. As a result, they risk injuring themselves or others if they are driving a car or operating dangerous equipment. Nevertheless, the findings of the study are bound to influence the care of many people with diabetes.

MYTH: People with diabetes can't eat normally, hold down a decent job, or do any of the other things healthy people do.

FACT: There's no reason that you cannot pursue a career, participate in sports, have children, and eat normally when you have diabetes. With the right information and guidance, and a commitment to take good care of yourself, you can do practically anything you want. You may even find that you take better care of yourself than you would have if you hadn't developed the disease.

Now that you have the facts, you'll want to know more about how to control your diabetes without letting it control you. But first, you should learn as much as you can about the disease itself—what it is, what causes it, and how it affects you.

CHAPTER 2

What Is Diabetes?

Diabetes mellitus (the medical term for diabetes) is a disorder related to your body's ability to use, or *metabolize*, the energy from the food you eat. It is caused by a deficiency of or an impairment in the action of *insulin*, a hormone secreted by the pancreas gland located just behind the stomach. Insulin helps your body's tissues store and use the sugars (glucose), protein, and fats circulating in your bloodstream after a meal.

To better understand the symptoms and complications that you may experience when you have diabetes, it helps to know how a person uses insulin and processes food. When you eat a meal, proteins, fats, and carbohydrates in your food are broken down in the small intestine into forms of energy your body can use: proteins are split into *amino acids* (the building blocks of proteins), fats are converted into fatty acids known as *triglycerides*, and carbohydrates are broken down into simple sugars, the most abundant of which is *glucose*. These nutrients are absorbed through the wall of the small intestine and into the bloodstream, where they are used to fuel all of your bodily functions, such as the movement of your muscles.

Glucose circulating in your blood is your body's primary source of energy, and is the main source of energy for your brain. In fact, glucose is so important that you body has developed a sophisticated system of checks and balances to ensure that your body's tissues—particularly your brain cells—get the right amount of sugar to function properly. (When blood sugar concentrations fall too low and the brain doesn't get enough sugar to function, a condition known as *hypoglycemia*, you may begin to feel irritable and lightheaded. If the problem isn't corrected, you could faint, or even experience convulsions. This is known as *hypoglycemic shock*.) Two of the major controls of this system are the hormones insulin and *glucagon*, both of which are secreted by specialized *islet* cells in the pancreas.

As blood sugar levels rise after a meal, they trigger the release of insulin from the *beta* islet cells in the pancreas. Once in your bloodstream, insulin is attracted to various cells in your body by *insulin receptors* on the surface of the cells in the same way that a magnet attracts a metal object. These receptors bind insulin to the cell, where it performs its main task: helping the cell soak up glucose from the bloodstream. With the help of insulin, your body's cells can absorb sugar ten times faster than without it. As the cells absorb glucose from the bloodstream, blood sugar levels go down.

When blood sugar concentrations fall, the pancreas stops secreting insulin and begins secreting the hormone glucagon. This hormone helps raise blood glucose levels between meals by triggering the release of sugars stored in the liver and proteins from muscle which the liver converts to sugar.

Food isn't the only thing that affects insulin production and blood sugar levels. Exercise can lower blood sugar levels, as glucose circulating in the bloodstream is used to fuel the working muscles. Such physical stresses as illness, surgery, or pregnancy can cause blood sugar levels to rise. Even everyday emotional upsets can raise blood sugar levels. Certain drugs can raise or lower blood sugar levels as well. Healthy people adjust to these daily fluctuations in blood sugar levels by secreting more or less insulin as needed, and blood sugar concentrations remain within safe levels—usually between 70 and 115 mg/dl (milligrams of sugar per deciliter [3 ounces] of blood; 100 mg is about 2/1000 of an ounce).

When you have diabetes, either your pancreas doesn't produce insulin or your body's tissues don't use insulin effectively. As a result, glucose builds up in the blood. In an effort to remove the excess sugar, the kidneys excrete large amounts of water and essential body elements, causing two of the typical symptoms of diabetes: frequent urination and increased thirst. Since the cells in the body are not getting a supply of glucose, the body turns to stored fat for energy. It also begins to take proteins from the muscles and converts them into sugar in the liver. Without insulin, however, the body cannot use these fuels either, and severely affected people with diabetes begin to lose weight. When the body tries to use fats for fuel, it breaks them down into products known as *ketones*. But without insulin, the body cannot use ketones. Instead, ketones build up in the bloodstream as acids, resulting in a condition known as *diabetic ketoacidosis*. If left untreated, diabetic ketoacidosis leads to coma and death.

Keeping your blood sugar levels under control through good eating habits, exercise, and, when necessary, the use of medication, is the best way to avoid symptoms and reduce the risk for the major complications associated with the disease. As you'll see in the chapters that follow, *most of the recommendations for staying healthy with diabetes are no different from those for people who do not have diabetes*.

Two Types of Diabetes

Diabetes is not one disease, but a group of disorders with one thing in common: abnormally high blood sugar levels. As mentioned in Chapter 1, there are two major forms of diabetes: insulin-dependent diabetes and non-insulin-dependent diabetes.

Insulin-dependent diabetes can develop at any age, but usually occurs in children or young adults, which is why it used to be called juvenile-onset diabetes. In this type of diabetes, the pancreas produces little or no insulin, and affected people must take insulin shots to survive; hence the name insulin-dependent diabetes.

Symptoms of insulin-dependent diabetes include frequent urination, excessive thirst, constant hunger (or sometimes loss of appetite, particularly in young children), blurred vision, and extreme fatigue. Because symptoms appear in a matter of days or weeks and are dramatic, most people with this type of diabetes are diagnosed within a month of the onset of symptoms.

Scientists still don't know what causes insulin-dependent diabetes. Research in the past twenty years, however, has tremendously increased our understanding of the disease. Scientists now know, for instance, that insulin-dependent diabetes is an *autoimmune disease;* that is, the body's immune defense system for some reason treats its own insulin-producing cells as if they were foreign. In people with insulin-dependent diabetes, the body mounts an immune system attack on these cells and destroys them.

Scientists have found that a cluster of genes that regulate the body's immune defense system, known as the *histocompatibility leukocyte antigen* (HLA) complex, is related to inheritance of insulin-dependent diabetes in some people. At least two HLA antigen types are associated with diabetes, and if you inherit one or both of them, there's a greater chance that you'll develop insulin-dependent diabetes. Inheriting one type of HLA antigen increases the risk of developing insulin-dependent diabetes three- to five-fold. When both types of HLA antigens are present, the risk increases ten- to twenty-fold over that of the general population.

But genes alone aren't enough to cause insulin-dependent diabetes. Studies involving identical twins, who share the same genes, have shown that when one twin develops insulin-dependent diabetes, the other twin develops the disease only 50 percent of the time. Apparently, you don't inherit the disease itself, but a tendency to get the disease. Scientists suspect that some outside influences—possibly one or more viruses or even certain drugs—may be needed to trigger the disease in susceptible people.

Once the autoimmune process is triggered, it may be months or even years before insulin production by the pancreas is affected. The only telltale sign at this stage is that most affected people have antibodies to islet cells or to their own insulin circulating in the bloodstream, which is extremely rare among people who do not develop diabetes.

Symptoms of insulin-dependent diabetes usually don't appear until 80 to 90 percent of the insulin-producing beta cells have already been destroyed. At this point, insulin levels in the bloodstream are low or undetectable.

Once treatment has begun, some people with insulin-dependent diabetes start producing insulin again. This is what is known as the *honeymoon phase*. During this time, the need for insulin shots may decrease dramatically. Some people may even be able to stop taking insulin altogether, although this may not be a good idea. There's some evidence to suggest that if you keep taking insulin during the honeymoon phase, it will be prolonged. The honeymoon phase can last for only a few weeks or for a year or more.

Insulin-dependent people have been described as having *unstable, labile,* or *brittle diabetes*. There is no precise medical definition of those terms, but the lives of those affected are constantly being disrupted by episodes of hypo- or hyperglycemia. Most specialists in diabetes do not consider this a type of diabetes, but rather, a reflection of management difficulties by the patient or family. These are often a result of emotional or social problems.

Thanks to our new understanding of insulin-dependent diabetes, novel approaches to treatment are being developed. One of the more promising developments involves the use of immunosuppressive drugs to halt the body's autoimmune attack on its own insulin-producing cells. Scientists have found, for instance, that *cyclosporine* (brand name Sandimmune), usually used to prevent rejection of a transplanted organ, preserves the function of insulin-producing beta cells for at least the first year after diabetes has been diagnosed. Another immunosuppressive drug, *azathioprine* (brand name Imuran), has been shown to reduce the severity of insulin-dependent diabetes when administered in the first three or four years after diagnosis.

Most of these studies involved people who already had symptoms of diabetes. But the destruction of beta cells by the immune system begins several years before the disease becomes apparent. For this reason, scientists at the University of Florida in Gainesville and elsewhere are trying to determine whether immunosuppressive therapy can prevent diabetes altogether in people at high risk of developing the disease. So far, twenty-four-year-old Peggy Polopolus, an actress in New York, is living proof that the new drug therapy works. Peggy was fourteen when her younger sister Eleni contracted insulin-dependent diabetes. Peggy then underwent a special blood test for antibodies to the islet cells that appear when the destructive process is going on. This test revealed that she was at risk of developing the disease as well. Two years later, when Peggy's blood sugar levels began to climb and her insulin levels began to fall—signaling that she was just months away from developing full-blown diabetes—Peggy began taking Imuran, which has been used for the past twenty-five years to prevent rejection of transplanted organs and to ease the pain of rheumatoid arthritis.

Ten years later at this writing, Peggy remains symptom-free. The success of her treatment has led researchers at the University of Florida, Harvard, the University of Washington—Seattle, and the University of Colorado to recruit some 10,000 close relatives of people with insulin-dependent diabetes so that the treatment can be tested on a larger scale.

Again, only about 5 to 10 percent of affected people have insulin-dependent diabetes. Most people have non-insulin-dependent diabetes. In this form of diabetes, the pancreas still produces some insulin, but often not enough to lower blood sugar levels. Moreover, the insulin that the body does produce isn't used efficiently, a condition known as *insulin resistance*.

While this type of diabetes can develop at any age, it is usually diagnosed after age forty, which is why it was formerly referred to as adult-onset or maturity-onset diabetes. Although some people with this form of diabetes may need to take insulin shots to control their blood sugar, or when they are acutely ill, they are not otherwise dependent on insulin shots to survive; hence the name non-insulin-dependent diabetes.

Symptoms of non-insulin-dependent diabetes may be vague. Some people may experience fatigue, frequent urination (particularly at night), unusual thirst, nearsightedness (myopia) or blurred vision, or a sudden weight loss. Wounds or infections of the gums, skin, and urinary tract may heal more slowly than usual. Women may notice itching in the genital area as a result of a yeast infection. (The yeast in the vagina thrive on the high sugar content of genital secretions.) Many people may have no symptoms at all, and the disease can go undiagnosed for years. Still others may mistake their symptoms for another medical problem; frequent urination, for instance, is also a symptom of a urinary tract infection. Sometimes the disease is diagnosed only after complications, such as heart disease or nerve damage, have developed. This is why regular medical checkups—including a simple blood sugar test—are a must.

No one knows yet how non-insulin-dependent diabetes develops. Scientists suspect that insulin resistance may be related to problems with *insulin receptors* on the surfaces of cells. As mentioned earlier, these receptors are specialized parts of a cell that attract and bind insulin to the cell. Unless insulin is bound to the cell, it can't help the cell process glucose.

A second possibility: for some reason, the complex process by which glucose enters the cell after insulin is bound to it becomes impaired. Indeed, new research suggests that these *postbinding problems* are primarily responsible for insulin resistance in most people with non-insulin-dependent diabetes. Scientists are now studying glucose absorption in individual cells to determine the exact cause of the problem.

While it's still not clear what causes insulin resistance, being overweight clearly contributes to the problem. Numerous studies have shown that weight gain uniformly leads to the development of insulin resistance in people of normal weight who previously had normal insulin sensitivity.

Insulin resistance in itself initially does not lead to high blood sugar levels. At first, the pancreas compensates by stepping up its production of insulin. Over time, however, the beta cells of the pancreas become overtaxed and produce less and less insulin. Blood sugar levels rise as a result, ultimately leading to the development of full-blown diabetes.

You may be at a greater risk of developing non-insulin-dependent diabetes if you are over age forty and overweight. In fact, in 1980, the Expert Committee on Diabetes of the World Health Organization singled out obesity as the most powerful risk factor for the disease. About 75 percent of people with non-insulin-dependent diabetes are overweight.

Non-insulin-dependent diabetes also appears to run in families. Although this type of diabetes is not related to the HLA antigens associated with insulin-dependent diabetes, studies involving identical twins show that if one twin develops non-insulin-dependent diabetes, there is a 90 to 100 percent chance that the other will, too. More evidence of a hereditary link comes from a form of non-insulin-dependent diabetes that often develops in childhood (maturity-onset diabetes of the young).

The good news is that the impaired insulin production and insulin resistance associated with non-insulin-dependent diabetes can be at least partially reversed. The prognosis is particularly good when the disease is diagnosed in its early stages. For many people, losing weight—even a little weight—is often all it takes to bring blood sugar levels down and keep diabetes in check.

In addition to the two major types of diabetes, there are a couple of other conditions associated with high blood sugar levels that may increase your risk of developing diabetes later on.

You may be diagnosed with *impaired glucose tolerance*, or IGT, if you have fasting blood sugar levels that are higher than normal (115 mg/dl or less) but lower than those used to diagnose diabetes mellitus (140 mg/dl or more). About 25 percent of people with IGT eventually develop diabetes. Sometimes IGT or diabetes occurs as a result of another illness, such as cystic fibrosis, chronic pancreatitis (inflammation of the pancreas) or other diseases of the pancreas, or Cushing syndrome and other hormonal disorders. Certain drugs may raise blood sugar levels as well, including the steroid prednisone, some antihypertensive medications, thiazide diuretics, estrogen-containing preparations, and psychoactive drugs.

Women who develop diabetes during pregnancy have what is known as *gestational diabetes*. (If you already had diabetes when you became pregnant, you don't have gestational diabetes.) This type of diabetes occurs in about 2 percent of all pregnant women, usually during the second or third trimester, when high levels of various hormones lead to insulin resistance. Most of the time, blood sugar levels return to normal after the baby is delivered. However, 30 to 40 percent of women with gestational diabetes will develop overt diabetes mellitus (usually non-insulin-dependent diabetes) within five to ten years.

Diagnosing Diabetes

In the near future, it may be possible to pinpoint those at highest risk of developing diabetes long before symptoms appear. Researchers at the University of Florida and elsewhere have developed blood tests to detect the presence of antibodies to islet cells or insulin among close relatives of people with insulin-dependent diabetes. As scientists learn more about the genetic links to diabetes, screening tests may become available to predict those at high risk near the time of birth, allowing them to take preventive measures right from the start. These tests are not yet practical enough for widespread use, however, and more evidence is needed before we can say that diabetes can be prevented.

In the meantime, physicians have several tests to diagnose diabetes. Your physician may recommend that you be tested for diabetes if you

- have a strong family history of diabetes
- are more than 20 percent over your desirable or ideal weight
- have given birth to a baby weighing more than nine pounds
- have had gestational diabetes
- have a history of recurrent skin, genital, or urinary tract infections
- are between the twenty-fourth and twenty-eighth weeks of pregnancy

Of course, you'll be advised to undergo diagnostic testing if you have any of the signs or symptoms of diabetes, such as increased urination or sugar in the urine. You may have to take a single test more than once, or take more than one of the following tests:

Random blood glucose test. This test involves having blood drawn from your arm, usually after a meal, to measure your blood glucose levels. Your doctor will diagnose diabetes if the blood glucose level is 200 mg/dl or more on two separate occasions.

Fasting blood glucose. This test involves having blood drawn from your arm after an overnight fast. Blood sugar levels below 115 mg/dl are considered normal. If blood sugar levels are greater than 115 mg/dl but less than 140 mg/dl, your doctor may recommend that you undergo a two-hour oral glucose tolerance test as well. Fasting blood sugar levels that are 140 mg/dl or higher on at least two separate occasions indicate that you have diabetes.

Oral glucose tolerance test. This test measures how the body responds to an increase in blood sugar after ingesting a high level of carbohydrates. During this test, blood glucose is measured before you have consumed a concentrated glucose drink, and again one and two hours later. Your doctor will diagnose diabetes if your blood sugar levels are 200 mg/dl or greater two hours after drinking the glucose *and* if your fasting blood glucose level is more than 140 mg/dl.

Your Health Care Team

Learning that you have diabetes can be an overwhelming experience. It's not unusual to feel isolated and a little frightened. You may be wondering how you are going to manage all by yourself. You need not—and *should not*—try to go it alone, particularly with the vast array of resources available to people with diabetes today. Start by familiarizing yourself with the professionals who can show you the ropes and help you adjust.

Of course, your doctor will be a key member of your treatment team. Should you see a specialist? Unless you have problems controlling your diabetes with the usual treatment, you are pregnant, or you have complications of diabetes, it's probably not necessary to see a diabetes specialist *(diabetologist)*. Your regular family physician, your internist (specialist in adult medicine), or your child's pediatrician, if your child is diagnosed with diabetes, will more than likely be able to provide most of the care needed. If your regular doctor believes that you or your child needs the care of a specialist, he or she will refer you to one.

Some people simply feel more comfortable under the care of a physician who specializes exclusively in the treatment of people with diabetes. If you *prefer* to seek out a specialist, ask your doctor, call local hospitals, or contact the American Diabetes Association or the National Institute of Diabetes and Digestive and Kidney Diseases for a referral to a diabetes specialist near you. (You'll find the addresses for these and numerous other helpful organizations in "Recommended Resources," beginning on page 187.) At any rate, you should designate one doctor as your *primary care physician*, the one you turn to first when problems arise.

Other members of your diabetes care team may include:

A diabetes educator: Learning all you can about diabetes is so important to good diabetes control that some physicians and clinics have developed educational programs devoted solely to educating patients and their families about diabetes. The people who implement these programs are known as diabetes educators, and they can be an invaluable part of your health care team. If your physician doesn't have a diabetes educator on his or her staff, the American Diabetes Association, which certifies educational programs that meet certain national standards, may be able to refer you to a diabetes educator or educational program in your area. (See page 187 for more information.)

A qualified nutritionist: If you have trouble making di-

etary changes on your own, this professional can help ease
you into more healthful eating habits. You should be aware
that in many states, no special license is required to give nutritional advice, so anyone can call himself or herself a nutritionist. You should find a qualified specialist in the treatment
of people with diabetes. Look for a professional who has a degree in nutrition from an accredited university, or preferably,
one who is a Registered Dietitian (R.D.). Your physician may
be able to provide you with a referral. Or contact a local university's nutrition department or a community hospital. The
American Dietetic Association will provide a list of Registered Dietitians in your area as well. For a referral, write to
the organization's National Center for Nutrition and Dietetics, 216 West Jackson Blvd., Suite 800, Chicago, IL
60606-6995, or call the American Dietetic Association's toll-
free consumer nutrition hotline: 1-800-366-1655.

An ophthalmologist: Because people with diabetes are at
risk of developing eye problems, routine eye examinations by
an eye doctor are recommended at least once a year for people over 30 and those age 12 to 30 years who have had diabetes for more than five years. If you have eye problems, you
may want to ask your physician for a referral to an ophthalmologist who specializes in and keeps up with the latest medical advances in the care of people with diabetes.

A podiatrist: If you develop foot problems, you may need
to see a foot specialist (podiatrist). Your doctor or your local
affiliate of the American Diabetes Association can provide
you with a referral.

A pharmacist: A good pharmacist does much more than
just dispense drugs. Look for one who keeps a patient
profile—a written record of drugs you have used, any dietary
restrictions, and any chronic conditions you may have. With
this information, your pharmacist can alert you to potential
drug or food-and-drug interactions that may occur with any
new prescriptions you have filled. Your pharmacist can also
provide you with information on storing drugs, saving money

with generic drugs, and taking medication properly. Many pharmacists can also assist with advice about and instructions for using such products as blood glucose monitors.

Your physician or friends may be able to provide you with a referral to a good pharmacist. Or contact your local affiliate of the American Diabetes Association.

A counselor or therapist: Changing old habits isn't always easy. And coping with the emotional ups and downs that often accompany a chronic illness like diabetes can be quite a challenge. (For more on making emotional adjustments, see Chapter 12.) A professional counselor can help make this period of adjustment easier, and can help you come to terms with your condition. Again, ask your physician for a referral to a therapist in your area.

Local support groups: People who share a common problem can be an enormous source of support. Consider joining a diabetes support group or, if you need to lose weight, such groups as Overeaters Anonymous or Weight Watchers. (You'll find a list of organizations that provide referrals to a variety of support groups in your area in the Appendix, beginning on page 187.)

With a strong health care team to back you, and with the help of this book, you'll learn how to manage your diabetes more effectively in your everyday life. Indeed, as you'll soon see, the most important member of your health care team is you.

Getting the Most from Your Diabetes Care Team

Because you are unique and your diabetes care plan must be tailored to your individual needs, no one book or pamphlet will be able to answer all of your questions. That is why it is essential to take advantage of the expertise of the people on your diabetes care team. To get the most out of your care team, try some of the suggestions here:

• Before your scheduled appointment, make a list of questions to ask your doctor, diabetes educator, or nutrition counselor. (You may want to carry a small notebook with you or write down your questions in your diabetes diary; see page 223 for a sample diary.) If your questions can't wait until your next office visit, call.

• If you don't understand the answer your doctor gives, ask him or her to explain it to you again in simpler terms. Then, to make sure you understand, repeat the answer in your own words to your doctor or other health care professional.

• Have your health care provider write down any instructions for you so that you will have something to refer to when you get home.

• Before you leave the office, check with your doctor about his or her availability, and see if there is someone else (the nurse or your diabetes educator, for instance) who can answer your questions when your physician is not around.

• Make sure you know how to do what is expected of you before you leave the doctor's office. Your doctor or diabetes educator will probably show you first, then have you perform the task by yourself.

• If you need help, ask. Studies have shown that people with plenty of support from family, friends, coworkers, and health care professionals are likely to take better care of themselves and have better control over their diabetes than people who don't have good social and medical support.

CHAPTER 3

Eating for Health and Diabetes Control

One of your biggest concerns after being told you have diabetes may be that you will have to go on a Spartan "diabetic diet" for the rest of your life. Healthy eating is still a mainstay in the management of both non-insulin-dependent diabetes and insulin-dependent diabetes. But during the past twenty years, major revisions have been made in the nutritional advice for people with diabetes. Today's meal plans are higher in complex carbohydrates and lower in protein and fat than those of years past. There's a more liberal attitude about sugar in your diet as well. *In fact, the nutritional guidelines for people with diabetes today are no different from those for healthy people without diabetes* recommended by the American Heart Association, the U.S. Dietary Guidelines for Americans, the National Research Council, and other national health organizations. This means you can look forward to meal plans that are more individualized, flexible, and *palatable* than ever before.

As you'll see in the pages to come, eating for health and diabetes control is common sense eating. There's no need to buy special dietetic foods; just choose regular, nutritious foods. (The only exceptions: you may want to buy no-fat, low-fat, and artificially sweetened foods to help control your weight and reduce your risk of heart disease.) For the most part, you can prepare the same foods for yourself that you prepare for your family and friends. In fact, by preparing wholesome, delicious, healthful meals for your family, you'll be instilling in them habits that will help keep them healthier, too.

Why What You Eat Is Important

If you have non-insulin-dependent diabetes, adopting healthy eating habits is one of the most important components of your diabetes care plan. Indeed, some people with non-insulin-dependent diabetes find that making a few dietary changes is all that's needed to keep blood sugar levels within a normal range. Your diet plays a major role in weight control, too, and if you have a weight management problem, losing even a little weight often improves blood glucose control. Even if you take diabetes medication, however, you should be aware that the drugs are not a substitute for good nutrition, but rather an adjunct to it. In fact, diabetes pills (oral hypoglycemic drugs) may stop working altogether if you don't eat properly.

Meal planning is an integral part of your diabetes care plan if you are insulin-dependent, as well, since the timing and dosage of your insulin and your blood sugar control will be affected by what and when you eat.

General Guidelines for Healthy Eating

There's no one formula for meal planning that works for all people with diabetes. So count on working closely with your doctor *and* a qualified dietitian or nutrition counselor in developing a meal plan suited to your needs, tastes, and preferences. (For information on finding a nutritionist, see page 189.) Your ultimate goal is to improve your current eating habits, which will in turn help improve your diabetes control. You can start by following a few common sense guidelines:

1. Learn which foods are the most nutrient-rich; that is, foods that are relatively high in carbohydrates, protein, vitamins and minerals, and low in fat.
2. Plan meals that contain foods from each of the four food groups (breads and cereals, fruits and vegetables, milk and dairy products, and meat and meat alternatives; see page 44).
3. Eat three balanced meals a day and on schedule, and have two or three snacks (as needed) on schedule.
4. Practice portion control in your serving sizes.
5. Exercise regularly (see Chapter 4).

Following is some basic information to help guide you in making wiser food choices when planning meals and snacks.

Calories

Your total food intake plays an important role in helping to manage your diabetes (and your weight, if needed), so meeting your body's calorie needs is the first consideration in planning your diet.

The total number of calories you need each day depends on your age, your height, your current weight, and your level of physical activity. You should work with your physician and

dietitian to determine your ideal body weight and total calorie intake.

If you are overweight (as are most people with non-insulin-
dependent diabetes), you will probably be advised to cut back
on your total calorie intake to lose weight. (You'll find more
tips on managing your weight beginning on page 46.) Many
people discover that simply cutting back on calories lowers
their blood sugar levels even before they lose a substantial
amount of weight.

If you are underweight or if you lost a considerable amount
of weight just before being diagnosed with diabetes, you may
have to increase your calorie intake to gain weight (or regain
weight you lost). Growing children and adolescents require
considerably more calories (relative to their size) than most
adults. During these years, children with diabetes and their
parents should plan with a dietitian or other health care team
member an appropriate set of guidelines based on the child's
food preferences and eating habits.

Pregnant women and breast-feeding mothers also need
more calories than usual. Your doctor or nutritionist can advise you of your increased calorie and nutrition needs during
pregnancy. (For more on nutrition during pregnancy, see
Chapter 9.)

Carbohydrates

Many people mistakenly think that people with diabetes
should avoid carbohydrates because these foods purportedly
raise blood sugar levels more quickly than protein or fat. You
may have also heard that carbohydrates are fattening and
should be avoided if you need to lose weight.

In fact, carbohydrates play a crucial role in healthy eating
and diabetes control—including weight management. To
make the best use of carbohydrates in your daily meal plans,
you'll need to know a little more about them.

Carbohydrates—the sugars and starches in foods—are the body's quickest source of energy. There are several different kinds of carbohydrates, some of which are more quickly converted into glucose in the bloodstream than others. In fact, scientists for many years now have been attempting to categorize carbohydrate-rich foods by how quickly they raise blood sugar levels, assigning a value or *glycemic index* to each food, in hopes of helping people with diabetes better manage their blood sugar levels. The problem is that each person is different and no two people respond to the same food in exactly the same way. You can, however, use the basic concept of the glycemic index to your advantage in your daily meal planning. Begin by learning about the different types of carbohydrates.

Refined sugars: These include cakes, cookies, candy bars, and other foods containing large amounts of refined sugar *(sucrose)*. These carbohydrates can cause blood sugar to rise and fall rapidly.

Simple sugars: These include fruits, fruit juices, and *fructose*, a sugar found naturally in fruit. Simple sugars can raise blood sugar levels quickly, which is why they are often recommended for the treatment of hypoglycemic reactions (see Chapter 7). Whole fruits also contain fiber, which slows the digestion of the sugar. (More on fiber below.)

Disaccharides: These are more complex sugars (also known as *lactose*, or milk sugar) found in milk and dairy products. Disaccharides take longer to break down in the body than fructose.

Complex carbohydrates: These are foods containing even more complex sugar molecules (known as *polysaccharides* or *starches)*, including whole-grain breads and cereals, pasta, potatoes, and beans and peas. The sugars in these foods take even longer for the body to break down into glucose.

Fiber: Dietary fiber—the indigestible part of plant foods—is not a carbohydrate, but it is present in all unrefined plant foods, such as vegetables, fruits, legumes, and grains, which happen to be the major sources of carbohydrates in our diets.

There are two types of dietary fiber: *water-insoluble fiber*, found in whole grains, vegetables, and the skins of fruits, and *water-soluble fiber*, found in oats and oat bran, fruits, and dried peas and beans. Experts have long known that insoluble fiber helps relieve constipation, prevents hemorrhoids, and may also help protect against colon cancer. More recently, researchers have suggested that soluble fiber may lower blood sugar levels among people with insulin-dependent diabetes and poorly controlled non-insulin-dependent diabetes. The fiber in these foods may help increase insulin sensitivity. Probably most important, soluble fiber has been found to lower blood cholesterol levels and, therefore, your risk of heart disease—but only when consumed as part of a low-fat diet.

Besides adding fiber to your diet, complex carbohydrates provide plenty of vitamins and minerals. Moreover, these foods are naturally low in fat (it's what you put on them that makes them fattening), so they are ideal for people who are watching their weight. In addition, eating plenty of high-fiber foods can increase feelings of fullness, helping you overcome the temptation to eat between meals.

Most experts now recommend that between 50 and 60 percent of your total calorie intake come from *complex carbohydrates*. So move over, meat. Make room for potatoes—and pasta, whole grain breads and cereals, dried peas and legumes, vegetables, and fruits with edible skins. (For more choices, see the table "High-Fiber Foods" which follows, and the bread/starch, fruit, and vegetable exchange lists beginning on page 206.) Choose foods containing unrefined carbohydrates with plenty of fiber rather than highly refined carbohydrates with a lower fiber content. In other words, it is better to eat an orange than drink a glass of orange juice. You should also select foods containing both soluble and insoluble fiber. But don't go overboard. Too much fiber can bind to and hinder the body's absorption of calcium and other minerals and vitamins, so limit yourself to no more than 25 to 30 grams of dietary fiber per day.

HIGH-FIBER FOODS

	Serving Portion	Total Fiber (grams)	Soluble Fiber (grams)
CEREALS			
All-Bran (Kellogg)	½ cup	12.9	2.1
Fiber One (General Mills)	½ cup	11.9	0.8
40% Bran Flakes	½ cup	4.3	0.3
Grape-Nuts (Post)	½ cup	5.6	1.6
Heartwise (Kellogg)	½ cup	2.8	1.4
Oat bran, cooked (Quaker)	¾ cup	4.0	2.2
Oat bran cereal, cold (Quaker)	¾ cup	2.9	1.5
Oatmeal, uncooked	⅓ cup	2.7	1.4
Raisin bran	¾ cup	5.3	0.9
Shredded wheat	⅔ cup	3.5	0.5
BREADS			
Bagel, plain	½ bagel	0.7	0.3
Pita bread	½ pocket	0.5	0.2
Pumpernickel bread	1 slice	2.7	1.2
White bread	1 slice	0.6	0.3
Whole-wheat bread	1 slice	1.5	0.3
FRUITS			
Apple, fresh (with skin)	1 medium	2.8	1.0
Blackberries, fresh	¾ cup	3.7	1.1
Cranberries, fresh	½ cup	1.6	0.5
Figs, dried	1½	2.3	1.1

Grapefruit, fresh	½ medium	1.4	0.9
Peaches, fresh (with skin)	1 medium	2.0	1.0
Pears, fresh (with skin)	1 small	2.9	1.1
Plums, red, fresh	2 medium	2.4	1.1
Prunes, stewed	¼ cup	1.6	0.9
Prunes, dried	3 medium	1.7	1.0
Raisins	2 tbsp.	0.4	0.2
Raspberries, fresh	1 cup	3.3	0.6
Strawberries, fresh	1¼ cup	1.8	0.6

VEGETABLES

Asparagus, cooked	½ cup	1.8	0.7
Beets, canned, cooked	½ cup	2.2	0.7
Broccoli, cooked	½ cup	2.4	1.2
Brussels sprouts, cooked	½ cup	3.8	2.0
Cabbage, fresh	1 cup	1.5	0.6
Carrots, sliced, cooked	½ cup	2.0	1.1
Carrots, fresh	1 medium	2.3	1.1
Cauliflower, cooked	½ cup	1.0	0.4
Corn, whole kernel, cooked	½ cup	1.6	0.2
Kale, cooked	½ cup	2.5	0.7
Okra, frozen, cooked	½ cup	4.1	1.0
Peas, green, frozen, cooked	½ cup	4.3	1.3
Potatoes, white, cooked (with skin)	½ cup	1.5	0.8
Spinach, cooked	½ cup	1.6	0.5
Sweet potato, cooked (flesh only)	⅓ cup	2.7	1.2
Zucchini, cooked	½ cup	1.2	0.5

LEGUMES
(DRIED PEAS AND BEANS)

Butter beans, cooked	½ cup	6.9	2.7
Chick-peas, cooked	½ cup	4.3	1.3
Kidney beans, cooked	½ cup	6.9	2.8

Lima beans, cooked	½ cup	4.3	1.1
Lentils, cooked	½ cup	5.2	0.6
Pinto beans, cooked	½ cup	5.9	1.9
Split peas, cooked	½ cup	3.1	1.1

Excerpted with permission from Anderson, James W., *Plant Fiber in Foods.* Lexington, Kentucky, HCF Nutrition Research Foundation, Inc., 1990. Copyright 1990 by James W. Anderson, M.D.

What about table sugar and other foods high in refined sugars? Although in the past, people with diabetes were advised to avoid sugar, scientists now recognize that a modest amount of table sugar eaten with other foods is not harmful and may actually help you follow your meal plan by making your diet more palatable and offering you a wider variety of food choices. Because of this new thinking, you may be permitted to eat small amounts of these foods as long as you eat them along with complex carbohydrates and protein, and space them out fairly evenly over the day.

There are, however, two important reasons to limit the amount of added sugar you eat. To begin with, the calories supplied by sugar and sweetened foods are largely "empty calories"; that is, the calories in these foods have little or no additional nutritive value. On the other hand, foods that naturally have sugar in them—whole fruits, for instance—contain carbohydrates, vitamins, minerals, and other nutrients, such as fiber. Second, many foods containing large amounts of added sugar, such as cakes, pies, cookies, ice cream, and sweet rolls, also contain a hefty amount of fat.

One way to cut back on sweets is simply to eat high-sugar foods less often and in smaller amounts. Another way is to replace table sugar with a sugar substitute, such as aspartame (NutraSweet, Equal), acesulfame (Sunett, Sweet One) or saccharin (Necta Sweet, Sucaryl, Sweeta, Sweet 'n Low, Sweet 10). Some people find that saccharin has a bitter aftertaste, and table-top forms of aspartame lose their sweetness when heated, so they generally can't be used in cooking. For these reasons, it is probably best to keep a variety of sweeteners on hand, so that if one doesn't suit a particular need, another will.

What about *fructose?* This simple sugar has the same amount of calories as sucrose (sixteen calories per teaspoon), but is somewhat sweeter, so you can use less. It is also a little less taxing on your blood sugar levels, since it is absorbed more slowly by the gastrointestinal tract. Fructose also has the same properties as sucrose when used in cooking. Fructose is available in a granulated form and a liquid form (high-fructose corn syrup).

Don't be fooled by products claiming to be "dietetic" or "diabetic." This doesn't mean that they can be eaten in unlimited quantities. Usually these terms mean that a sugar substitute or sugar alcohol *(sorbitol)* has been used to sweeten the product and the total number of calories has been reduced as a result. Sometimes, however, the total calories in the "diabetic" food are the same (since sorbitol is a nutrient that contains calories) or higher as a result of more fat. Most experts now agree that the *fat* in sweets should be of greater concern to you than the sugar. Be sure to check the fat and calorie content of dietetic or diabetic products before you buy them. Check the price of the product, too; they often cost more than regular foods. Generally speaking, no diet needs these foods, which simply do not provide much value for their cost.

Protein

Protein in your diet supplies your body with the nine essential amino acids (building blocks of proteins) that it can't make on its own. But you don't need to eat a lot of protein to meet your daily requirement; protein from animal or plant sources should comprise from 12 to 24 percent of your total daily calorie needs. Most Americans easily consume much more protein than this.

Two three-ounce servings of lean red meat, poultry, or fish, together with protein from milk or milk products is all most average adults need each day. (Children and adolescents may need more protein during periods of growth; people with kidney damage may need less; check with your physician or nutritionist to determine your individual protein needs.)

To meet your protein need, choose foods high in protein but low in total fat (including saturated fat and cholesterol; for more on fat, see below). Fish, lean red meats, poultry (chicken and turkey) with the skin removed, and skim or low-fat milk and dairy products are good protein sources. Legumes, lentils and dried peas are excellent sources of protein without the fat (provided you cook them without fat drippings; see page 35 for cooking suggestions).

Fat

Although fat-rich foods are some of the most delicious, gram for gram they are more than twice as high in calories as carbohydrates and proteins: one gram of fat contains nine calories, compared to four calories per gram of protein or carbohydrate. There's some evidence to suggest that fat calories are simply more fattening than calories from other foods; that is, dietary fat is much more likely than other foods to be stored in your body's fat tissues. So you can see that if you have a weight problem, cutting back on dietary fat is one of the most effective ways you have of reducing calories and losing weight. But there's another good reason for *all* people with diabetes to control their fat intake: diets high in total fat, saturated fat, and cholesterol are associated with a higher risk of heart disease. Since you are already at a somewhat greater risk of developing heart disease by virtue of having diabetes (see page 115), you certainly don't need a high-fat diet contributing to your risk.

Because dietary fat contributes to obesity and heart disease, the American Diabetes Association and other national health organizations now advise people with diabetes to limit their *total fat* consumption to no more than 30 percent of their total daily calories. Twenty percent of these calories should come from *polyunsaturated* and *monounsaturated* fats. Polyunsaturated fats include liquid vegetable oils, such as corn oil, safflower oil, sunflower oil, sesame seed oil, and cottonseed oil. (The only exceptions are coconut oil and palm oil, which should be avoided as much as possible because they are high in saturated fat.) Olive oil and peanut oil are monounsaturated oils.

The remaining 10 percent of total fat may come from *saturated fats*, found in meat and dairy products. You should limit *cholesterol*, a fatty substance found in meat, dairy products, and eggs, to no more than 300 milligrams per day.

If all this sounds confusing, relax. There are a few fairly simple methods for reducing the fat and cholesterol in your diet. One of the easiest is to cut back on the foods highest in fat: meat and dairy products. Since these foods are also important sources of protein, vitamins, and minerals, it is not necessary to cut them out of your diet altogether. Instead, trY some of the following suggestions:

Reduce your intake of red meats (beef, lamb, pork, and veal). You can do this by limiting your serving size to three ounces (the size of a deck of playing cards), and eating these foods three times per week or less. When you do eat red meat, choose "select" and "choice" grades of red meat over "prime" meats, which contain the most fat, and cut off any visible fat before cooking. Use the meat exchange list on page 209 as a guide for making low-fat supermarket selections.

Increase your intake of poultry (chicken and turkey). Be sure to remove the skin from poultry before eating it, and use the white meat instead of the dark meat.

Increase your intake of fish. Fish is an excellent low-fat alternative to red meat, so try to increase your consumption of fish to two to three times per week. Limit your consumption of shellfish to once a week, however, as some shellfish tends to be high in cholesterol. Serving sizes of shellfish are important, too. One serving is equal to one lobster or crab, or six shrimp, oysters, scallops, or clams.

Increase your intake of legumes. Lentils, chick-peas, split peas, black-eyed peas, navy beans, kidney beans, black beans and other dried peas and beans are excellent substitutes for red meat, as they are high in carbohydrates, protein, vitamins, and iron, and low in fat. To help reduce intestinal gas, soak beans overnight in water with ⅛ teaspoon of baking soda per quart of water. Drain beans in the morning, add fresh water and seasonings (use herbs and spices instead of pork fat or fat drippings) and cook until done.

Reduce your intake of egg yolks and other high-cholesterol foods. Limit your use of egg yolks to three times per week (including in cooking). When cooking, the following can be substituted for one medium egg: two egg whites or ¼ cup of liquid, frozen or powdered egg substitute (such as Eggbeaters).

Other foods high in cholesterol include butter and other whole dairy products, red meats, and organ meats (liver, kidneys, brains, tongue).

Choose low-fat or skim milk and dairy products. You will reduce your fat intake by a sizeable amount simply by substituting low-fat and skim milk and dairy products for whole milk products. For instance, an 8-ounce glass of skim milk contains just trace amounts of fat, compared to 8 grams of fat in an 8-ounce glass of whole milk.

Use polyunsaturated and monounsaturated oils instead of saturated fats when cooking. Polyunsaturated oils include liquid corn, safflower, sunflower, and cottonseed oils. (Avoid the use of coconut and palm oils, which contain a high amount of saturated fat.) Monounsaturated oils include olive and peanut

oils. Use liquid or whipped margarine instead of stick margarine or butter.

Use reduced-fat cooking methods. Trim all visible fat from
the meats you buy and remove the skin from chicken before
cooking. Baking, poaching, broiling, roasting, stir-frying, and
stewing meats require the least amount of fat. Cook meat on
a rack so that the fat drips down. Avoid pan-frying or deep-
frying foods.

Eat smaller portions of fatty foods. Most experts now recommend smaller, three-ounce portions of meat, rather than
the six- to twelve-ounce portions you may be used to seeing
on your plate. A three-ounce portion is about the size of a
deck of playing cards.

Avoid cream sauces and creamy salad dressings. Try
lemon juice and herbs on vegetables instead. Use vinegar and
oil, lemon juice and oil, seasoned rice vinegar, mustard vinai-
grette, or other low-fat dressings on salads. Decrease your
use of sauces made with heavy cream and whole milk.

Should You Become a Vegetarian?

Many people find that avoiding meat altogether is one of
the easiest ways to reduce the fat and cholesterol in their
diets. There are several different ways of practicing vegetarianism: semi-vegetarians occasionally eat fish and poultry; *lacto-ovo vegetarians* include milk, dairy products, and
eggs but no meat in their diets: *lacto-vegetarians*, consume
milk and dairy products but no meat or eggs; *vegans* ex-
clude all meat, eggs, and dairy products from their diets.

Although vegetarian diets overall are considered to be
healthy (most vegetarians are closer to a healthy body
weight, have lower blood pressure, and a lower incidence of
heart disease, constipation and diverticular disease, and
cancer than nonvegetarians), there are some potential nutritional problems with vegetarianism, most of which can be
resolved with careful meal planning.

The first consideration is assuring that you get the full complement of nine essential amino acids your body needs from your diet to function properly. Unlike protein from animal products, which supply most or all of the nine amino acids, protein from vegetables is "incomplete," that is, it doesn't contain all of the nine essential amino acids. This means you will have to eat vegetable proteins with other vegetables and/or whole grains (for instance, peanut butter on whole-grain bread with a glass of skim milk), which is known as *mutual supplementation.* If you include milk and dairy products in your diet, this usually isn't a problem, since these foods supply most or all of the amino acids your body needs.

Another concern will be to avoid nutritional deficiencies, especially in calcium, vitamin B_{12}, and iron. Semi-vegetarians and lacto-ovo vegetarians are least likely to develop calcium and vitamin B_{12} deficiencies, since milk and dairy products usually supply adequate amounts of calcium and vitamin B_{12}. Getting enough iron may still be a problem for non-meat-eaters, however, since the iron in vegetables is not as readily absorbed by the body as the iron in meats. (To increase absorption of iron, eat iron rich foods, such as lentils and dried fruits, along with foods high in vitamin C, such as orange juice, tomatoes, or broccoli.)

Vegans are most vulnerable to developing nutritional deficiencies. In fact, most experts agree that it is impossible for people to meet all their nutritional needs on a strict vegan diet. For this reason, vegan diets are not recommended for children and women in their childbearing years. If you do try this extreme form of vegetarianism, you really must take supplements to avoid nutritional deficiencies.

A more precise way to reduce the fat in your diet is to keep track of your daily fat consumption by counting fat grams in the same way that you would count calories on a weight-reducing diet. First, you'll need to determine your total daily allowance of fat in grams (ask your dietitian or doctor to help). The average adult on a daily diet of 2,000 calories, with 30 percent of the calories from fat, should consume no more than 66 grams of fat per day.

Next, simply count the grams of fat in the foods you eat in the course of a day. If you go this route, you will have to become an avid label reader. Since it is not yet mandatory for manufacturers to list the nutritional content of a food on the label (new regulations now in the works by the U.S. Food and Drug Administration may soon require this), and since many fresh foods that you prepare yourself don't have labels, you may want to invest in a book that lists the fat and cholesterol content of various foods. (See page 193 for a few recommendations.) When counting fat grams, don't forget to include the pat of margarine you spread on your toast, the cooking oil you use to sauté your chicken breast, and the salad dressing you dribble over your greens.

You'll also need to know how to determine the fat content of foods you prepare for yourself. Basically, this involves adding up *all* of the fat in the individual ingredients and dividing by the number of servings the recipe yields. Your nutrition counselor can help you. Using the Food Exchange Lists beginning on page 206 simplifies matters, too. Here's an example, using tuna salad:

Ingredient	Fat Grams
one 6-ounce can of white tuna (water packed)	3
one tablespoon reduced-calorie mayonnaise	50
TOTAL FAT	53

53 fat grams ÷ three 2-ounce servings = 17.6 grams per 2-ounce serving

When shopping, be aware that it's not always enough to choose products whose labels claim that they are low in fat or cholesterol. Current food labeling regulations allow manufacturers to make such claims even though, for example, a low-cholesterol product may contain a substantial amount of saturated fat, which can raise your blood cholesterol level and your risk of heart disease. Some products claiming to be, say, "88 percent fat free," make such claims based on the weight or volume of the product, while the percentage of calories from fat ("fat calories") is still quite high. New, stricter labeling regulations are in the works to remedy these problems. In the meantime, when buying processed foods, you should learn how to calculate the percentage of calories from fat in a given product.

Here's a simple formula for calculating the percentage of calories that come from fat: Multiply the grams of fat per serving by 9 (the number of calories in one gram of fat). Then divide that number by the total number of calories in a serving, and multiply by 100.

Here's an example using a serving of canned beef ravioli in tomato sauce containing 6 grams of fat and 180 calories per serving:

$$
\begin{aligned}
& 6 \quad \text{(grams of fat per serving)} \\
\times\ & 9 \quad \text{(calories in one gram of fat)} \\
=\ & 54 \quad \text{(fat calories)} \\
\div\ & 180 \quad \text{(total calories)} \\
=\ & .30 \\
\times\ & 100 \\
=\ & 30 \quad \text{(percentage of calories from fat)}
\end{aligned}
$$

Sodium

Sodium is a major component of table salt. When eaten in excessive amounts, sodium can cause some people's blood pressure to rise. Since people with diabetes are more likely to have high blood pressure than people who don't have diabetes, and since high blood pressure is a major risk factor for heart disease, kidney damage, and stroke, you can see why it makes sense to limit your consumption of sodium.

Your body needs a certain amount of sodium to maintain blood volume and fluid balance, to help exchange nutrients and wastes across the cell walls, and to aid in the transmission of nerve impulses. The U.S. Dietary Guidelines for Americans recommend that you consume no more than 3,000 to 4,000 milligrams (3 to 4 grams) of sodium per day. Most Americans consume from 5,000 to 10,000 milligrams of sodium per day.

You will definitely be advised to cut back on sodium if you already have high blood pressure or kidney damage. Even if you don't have high blood pressure or kidney problems, it's a good idea to reduce your sodium intake. You can do this by following a no-added-salt diet; that is, you should use moderation when cooking with salt, or better yet, substitute herbs and spices for salt when cooking. You should also replace the salt shaker on your table with an herbal blend, pepper, lite-salt (which has half the sodium of regular table salt) or a salt substitute (except if you have kidney problems; the potassium in salt substitutes can be just as damaging to the kidneys as sodium). Rinse salty foods whenever possible. You should also reduce your use of canned, boxed, or frozen prepared meals, as well as fast foods. These are usually loaded with sodium. If you do buy processed foods, look for low-salt or no-salt versions.

Vitamins and Minerals

There's no evidence that people with diabetes have any greater need for vitamins and minerals than the general population. If you eat a variety and balance of foods, including plenty of fresh fruits and vegetables, you will invariably meet your daily need for most vitamins and minerals, and you won't need to take vitamin pills.

If a medical evaluation reveals that you have a vitamin or mineral deficiency, you will probably be advised to increase your food intake to correct the problem. Food naturally contains nutrients that vitamin and mineral supplements are lacking.

If you are on a weight-management program and your calorie intake is restricted to fewer than 1,200 calories per day, your doctor or nutritionist will probably advise that you take a multivitamin supplement, since it is almost impossible to meet 100 percent of the recommended dietary allowances on such a restricted diet. Pregnant women and nursing mothers will also be given a special prenatal supplement. And if your calcium intake from food is less than 800 milligrams per day, a calcium supplement may be recommended.

Water

Although there are no recommended dietary allowances for water, it is the body's most vital component. Some 55 to 60 percent of an adult's body weight—and an even higher percentage of a child's weight—is water. Water and other body fluids are crucial in transporting nutrients to all the cells in your body and carrying away wastes. Drinking plenty of water is especially important when your diabetes is not under control, since high blood sugar levels can cause you to lose water and become dehydrated.

The amount of water you need depends on your level of activity, environmental conditions, and whether or not you are sick. Water and other beverages obviously help meet your daily need. The advantage of drinking water as opposed to other beverages, such as juices or regular soft drinks, is that water has zero calories and does not raise your blood sugar levels like juices or sugar-containing soft-drinks. Nearly all foods contain water, too. Most fruits and vegetables are up to 90 percent water; meats and cheeses contain at least 50 percent. But the water supplied by food is not enough to meet your body's daily need for water. To ensure an adequate fluid intake, try to drink four to six glasses of water every day.

What About Alcohol?

There's no nutritional reason to abstain completely from alcohol if you have diabetes, but you will need to make provisions for alcoholic beverages in your meal plan. Moderation is the key. Two ounces of alcohol one or two times a week is a prudent amount. Since the calories in alcohol have no other nutritional value (empty calories!), most experts recommend that you account for those calories by reducing your fat intake by a comparable amount (see "Exchange Values for Alcoholic Beverages," which follows). You should avoid sweetened alcoholic mixed drinks, liqueurs, and after-dinner drinks because of their increased sugar content.

Before you imbibe, you should be aware of the potential problems with alcohol consumption for people with diabetes. Alcohol is broken down in the liver, where it blocks the ability of the liver to make glucose. This is such a powerful effect that it can cause severe hypoglycemia in people without diabetes who drink on an empty stomach. For people with diabetes, particularly those who take insulin or diabetes pills, alcohol is especially dangerous if it is not taken with food. So whenever you drink, *always* eat something first.

You should also be aware that when you drink, you and those around you may find it harder to recognize the early warning signs of hypoglycemia or to distinguish them from drunkenness. (For more on recognizing and treating hypoglycemia, see Chapter 7.) You will also find it more difficult to follow your management plan if you are intoxicated. One way to lessen these effects of alcohol is to drink slowly. Take one drink and nurse it all night.

Finally, alcohol can raise blood triglycerides, and high triglycerides have been associated with an increased risk of heart disease. In fact, if you have been diagnosed with *hypertriglyceridemia* (high blood triglycerides), your physician may recommend that you abstain from drinking alcoholic beverages altogether. You should also avoid alcohol if your blood glucose is out of control, you are attempting to lose weight, or you are pregnant or trying to become pregnant.

Exchange Values for Alcoholic Beverages

Item	Average Serving (oz.)	Alcohol (gram/serving)	Calories per Serving	Exchange Values
Beer (regular)	12	13.0	151	2 fats and 1 starch
Beer (light)	12	10.1	97	2 fats
Table wine				
Red	4	11.6	83	2 fats
White	4	11.6	80	2 fats
Distilled spirits (86 proof gin, whiskey, rum, vodka, scotch)	1.5	15.3	107	2 fats

Why When You Eat May Be as Important as What You Eat

If you take insulin or diabetes pills, *when* you eat your meals can be as important as *what* you eat. Injected insulin and oral medications work constantly to lower blood sugar. Spreading food out evenly throughout the day helps to balance the effect of these drugs and keep blood sugar levels from dropping too low. If you take insulin, a midafternoon snack may be needed and a bedtime snack will probably be recommended to ensure that your blood sugar concentrations don't fall too low during the night.

Eating regularly helps if you are trying to lose weight, too. By eating three meals at planned times throughout the day, you are less likely to get hungry and will be more able to control what you eat. Because it is harder to control your eating when you're hungry, skipping meals may ultimately make it more difficult to lose weight.

Generally speaking, you should try to spread your calories as evenly as possible over your major daily meals. You should avoid a large concentration of calories at any one meal, which might overwhelm your already reduced ability to process food.

Food Exchanges and Other Meal-Planning Systems

A number of meal-planning systems have been developed to help make healthful eating easier for you. Some of the easiest and most widely used are food group plans. These plans help you eat balanced meals by sorting foods of similar origin and nutrient content into groups and specifying how many servings from each group you should eat. The most familiar of these is the Four Food Group Plan. The four food groups are 1) fruits and vegetables, 2) breads and cereals, 3) milk and milk products, and 4) meat and meat alternatives (including poultry, fish, and legumes). For an adult, the recommended number of daily servings are as follows:

- four servings of vegetables and fruits
- four servings of breads and cereals

- two servings of milk and milk products
- two servings of meat and meat alternatives

If you use the Four Food Group Plan, be sure to choose *low-fat* foods from each group (whole grain breads instead of croissants or biscuits; skim or low-fat milk and ice milk instead of whole milk and ice cream; fish and chicken with skin removed instead of hot dogs and hamburgers). Using the Four Food Group Plan *doesn't* mean you can eat unlimited quantities of these foods, either. When using this meal planning system, you will have to pay attention to serving sizes and practice portion control. Here are some guidelines for each of the four food groups:

Fruits and vegetables: One serving equals 1 medium apple, banana, or orange, ½ grapefruit, 1 melon wedge; ¾ cup juice; ½ cup berries; ½ cup diced, cooked, or canned fruit; ¼ cup dried fruit; ½ cup cooked or raw vegetables; 1 cup leafy raw vegetables; ½ cup cooked legumes; ¾ cup vegetable juice.

Breads and cereals: One serving equals 1 slice of bread; ½ cup cooked cereal, rice, or pasta; one ounce of ready-to-eat cereal; ½ bun, bagel, or English muffin; 1 small roll, biscuit, or muffin; three to four small or two large crackers.

Milk and milk products: One serving equals 1 cup milk or yogurt; two ounces processed cheese food; one and one-half ounces cheese.

Meat and meat alternatives: One serving equals two to three ounces lean, cooked meat, poultry or fish (total five to seven ounces per day); for meat alternatives, count one egg, ½ cup cooked legumes, or 2 tablespoons peanut butter as one ounce of meat (about ⅓ serving).

Another widely used meal planning system is the food exchange system, developed by the American Diabetes Association, the American Dietetic Association, and the U.S. Public Health Service. An *exchange* is a serving of food in a specific amount from a particular list. It can be substituted for any other food *on the same list*. Each exchange is approximately equal in number of calories and in amount of carbohydrate, protein, fat, vitamins, minerals, and fiber. There are six exchange lists: the bread/starch exchange list, the meat exchange list, the vegetable exchange list, the fruit exchange list, the milk exchange list, and the fat exchange list. (See page 206.)

When using the exchange system, keep in mind that while the types of food you eat are important, the *amount* of food you eat is also very important. Your dietitian will teach you how many choices to make from each list at each meal. Be sure to check with your nutrition counselor about foods or recipes that you love but that are not on your exchange list. Often, these can be worked into your meal plan as occasional treats, either as is or slightly modified.

Special Circumstances

If You Need to Lose Weight

As we have already said, if you have non-insulin-dependent diabetes, one of the single most important things you can do to control your diabetes is to lose weight. But what's the best way to lose weight? A sensible, low-fat eating plan, along with regular exercise, is the safest way for most people with diabetes. You may find that once you begin following your diabetes care plan, making more nutritious *low-fat* food choices, and increasing your level of activity, you will lose weight without even trying. Most people will, however, have to make a concerted effort to get the weight off and an even bigger effort to keep it off.

Start by setting sensible goals, beginning with a determination of what you *should* weigh. Compare your current weight with the "ideal" weight for your height in the standard height and weight tables on page 205. Keep in mind, however, that these are "suggested" weights for the average person. Not everybody will—or can—conform to the norm, no matter how hard he or she tries. Be sure to discuss what your ideal weight should be with your doctor or nutritionist to ensure that you have set a realistic goal for yourself.

Next, develop a reasonable time frame within which to lose the weight. A good rule of thumb is to plan to lose between one and two pounds per week. By gradually losing weight this way, you will be more likely to shed unwanted fat instead of muscle. By losing at a slow and steady pace, you will also be more likely to keep the weight off for good.

Your doctor or nutritionist can also help determine how much you should eat to achieve your goals. Since most weight problems are caused by eating more calories than you expend, weight loss can be achieved by creating a calorie deficit, in which you take in fewer calories than you expend. You can do this by eating fewer calories, increasing your level of physical activity, or both. Most adults can lose weight on a 1,200-calorie-per-day diet. Don't try to speed things up by eating even less or by skipping meals or between-meal snacks, particularly if you take insulin or oral diabetes medication. Doing so can lead to dangerous bouts of hypoglycemia, can compromise you nutritionally, and can prompt you to binge later on to make up for the meal or snack you missed. Losing weight too rapidly can also lead to dangerous electrolyte (mineral) imbalances. In fact, you should *never* restrict your food intake to less than 1,200 calories per day unless you are under a doctor's supervision. You should also avoid fad diets that emphasize one food or food group to the exclusion of others, such as "high protein," or "grapefruit" diets; these diets almost always cause nutritional deficiencies and can lead to dangerous mineral imbalances. Moreover, the diets don't teach you to practice good eating habits. After the diet is over and you resume your normal eating habits, the weight usually comes right back on.

One of the easiest ways to cut calories is to cut out the most calorie-rich foods in your diet: fats. Replace fatty foods with high-carbohydrate, high-fiber foods, particularly complex carbohydrates, such as breads and cereals made from whole grains, and dried peas and beans. These foods are naturally high in vitamins and low in fat. And as we pointed out earlier, the fiber in complex carbohydrates increases feelings of fullness, possibly helping you resist the temptation to eat.

For those who want a structured weight-loss program that includes the support of others, Weight Watchers is one of the most successful. The program offers several sensible meal plans and weekly support sessions in which group members discuss their mutual problems. Other popular programs based on group therapy are TOPS ("Taking Off Pounds Sensibly") and Overeaters Anonymous. (See page 190 for addresses.) Remember, though, that these programs are designed for people who don't have diabetes. If you do participate in a structured weight-loss program, be sure to keep in close touch with your doctor, as your need for oral medication or insulin may change as you lose weight.

What about over-the-counter diet pills, such as Acutrim, Control, Dexatrim, and Diadex? These products are not recommended for people with diabetes because the active ingredient in them, *phenylpropanolamide*, may raise your blood sugar levels. They also have other undesirable side effects, and their effectiveness as diet aids is questionable.

If you are moderately obese (more than twenty-five pounds overweight), your fasting blood sugar levels are dangerously high, and you and your doctor are in a hurry to see results, he or she may recommend that you go on a nutritionally balanced, very-low-calorie diet. These diets, which are really modified fasts during which you consume enough protein and nutrients to keep you healthy, usually involve drinking specially formulated high-protein shakes instead of eating food and taking a daily vitamin and mineral supplement.

These diets are much safer than the high-protein diets developed in the mid- to late 1970s, which were associated with a number of deaths in the United States. But they're not for everybody. And they're not without risks, including dehydration, electrolyte imbalances, postural hypotension (low blood pressure when you stand up), and increased uric acid concentrations, which could lead to gout. These complications can be quickly identified and readily managed by your physician, which is why *you must be under close medical supervision for the duration of the diet.*

A doctor's supervision is particularly important during "refeeding," the period in which you are reintroduced to solid foods. Too much food after severe calorie restrictions can lead to *cardiac arrhythmias* (abnormal heart rhythms). Indeed, many of the deaths associated with liquid-protein diets in the 1970s occurred within the two-week period when the dieters stopped their consumption of liquid protein and returned to conventional foods.

Because of the risks associated with very-low-calorie diets, you should not attempt to use similar over-the-counter weight-loss products, such as Ultra Slim-Fast, *unless you have the approval of your doctor and are closely monitored.*

For people who are more than 100 pounds overweight and who fail repeatedly to lose weight using very-low-calorie diets and other methods, "stomach stapling" or bypass surgery may be an option. The procedure involves having a surgeon create a smaller stomach pouch with a row of surgical staples or create a new stomach outlet that bypasses most of the small intestine. Your doctor can tell you whether you are a candidate for this type of surgery, and discuss the risks of such an operation.

No matter what method you use to reduce your daily intake of calories from food, you should also plan to increase your daily expenditure of calories through exercise. Regular exercise helps you burn calories and fat and helps you retain vital muscle mass. Because you are increasing your calorie expenditure through exercise, you may find that you don't have to cut your daily calorie consumption as much as when you merely diet. In this way, you may feel less deprived, and may be less likely to go off your diet. (To find out how to start an exercise program, see Chapter 4.)

After you have lost weight, the greater challenge is often keeping excess weight off for good. This means changing your eating and exercise habits, not just for a few weeks, but for the rest of your life. For this reason, behavior modification—techniques that help you change old habits—is a must for anyone who is serious about losing weight. If you are losing weight with the help of your doctor, a dietitian, or one of the structured weight-loss programs mentioned earlier, these professionals can offer individual or group counseling to help you identify and change some of the habits that may have contributed to your weight problem in the first place. You should also enlist the support of your family and friends. You may want to try some of these techniques as well:

• Become more aware of your eating habits. For a week or two, keep a daily record of the foods you eat and the circumstances that encourage eating. For instance, do you tend to eat snacks while watching television? Do you eat to calm down after having an argument with your spouse or partner? Once you know what stimulates you to eat, you can work to eliminate those triggers.

• Keep food out of sight. Having food in plain view can act as a constant reminder to "eat, eat, eat." To help you resist temptation, store *all* foods behind closed doors—in the cupboard, pantry, or refrigerator.

• Keep candy and cookies out of the house. Don't even buy these foods when you are grocery shopping.

• Keep on hand plenty of low-calorie, high-fiber vegetables, such as carrots, broccoli, cauliflower, and celery, and strategically place them at the front of the refrigerator.

• Avoid eating while watching television or reading.

• Eat in one place—no matter what you are eating.

• Prepare a full table setting every time you eat. This helps slow the act of eating.

• Use smaller plates.

• Count each mouthful and place your utensils on your plate after every third mouthful.

You may want to set up a system in which you award yourself points for sticking with your diet. After successfully accumulating a certain number of points, reward yourself with money, a gift, or a vacation.

If you don't succeed in reaching your ideal weight, don't view your efforts as a total loss and stop trying altogether. Studies have shown that people who lose as little as ten to fifteen pounds often see major improvements in their blood glucose levels. So keep up the good work.

Eating Out

You have the most control over what you eat when you prepare your meals yourself. But having diabetes doesn't mean you can never eat at a friend's house or dine out. In fact, eating out is easier than ever today, thanks to the push by so many national health organizations and the demand by health-conscious consumers for restaurants to lighten up their menus. Even most fast-food restaurants offer leaner fare, including low-fat milk, burgers, and salads.

You will have to give some thought to what you order in a restaurant and to how much you should eat. According to Mayer B. Davidson, M.D., director of the diabetes program at Cedars-Sinai Medical Center in Los Angeles, you should make a habit of measuring foods at home so you'll be a better judge of portions you are served when eating out. If a serving is too large, eat only the amount allowed and take the rest home in a doggy bag. Before ordering, ask the server what is in the dish and how it is prepared. Dr. Davidson recommends that you use the following guidelines when ordering from the menu.

Order More Often	*Avoid*
Appetizers	
Tomato or vegetable juice, clear broth, raw vegetables, plain meat and fish, broth-based soups, fresh soup	Creamed soups, crackers, chips, dips, nuts, marinated and fried vegetables
Salads	
Fresh vegetables and fruit salads without dressing (request that dressing be served in a separate dish)	Salads with dressings added, molded salads, cheese mixtures
Meat, Fish, Poultry	
Lean cuts that are roasted, baked, broiled, or charcoal-grilled	Any that are fried, breaded, sautéed, or creamed in sauces or gravies
Eggs	
Soft, hard-boiled, or poached	Fried or scrambled

Sandwiches

Lean meats, low-fat cheeses, water-packed fish, low-fat cold cuts

Regular cold cuts, brisket, sausage, corned beef, pastrami, hot dogs, fatty hamburgers, cheese, sandwiches grilled in fat, oil-packed meats and fish

Vegetables

Any stewed, steamed, boiled, baked, or raw

Creamed, escalloped, au gratin, fried, sautéed, in sauces

Potatoes, Rice, Noodles

Baked, mashed, boiled, or steamed

Fried, creamed, escalloped, in sauces

Breads and Cereals

Hard or soft rolls, bagels, English muffins, crackers made without fat, hot and cold cereals made without fat, tortillas, air-popped popcorn

Sweet rolls, coffee cakes, pastries, nut and fruit breads, doughnuts, muffins made with fat, cakes, cookies, pies, crackers made with fat, oil-popped popcorn

Fats

Margarine, light or diet margarine, oil-based or light or diet salad dressings, light mayonnaise, light sour cream, light cream cheese

Gravy, fried foods, cream sauces, creamy salad dressings, bacon, sausage, cream cheese, sour cream, butter, tartar sauce

Desserts

Fresh fruit, sherbet, fat-free ice cream, angel food cake, sugar-free Jell-O, nonfat yogurt	Sweetened fruits, custards, puddings, pies, cakes, cookies, candy, chocolate, pastry

Beverages

Coffee, tea, diet soda, plain or carbonated water, sugar-free beverages	Chocolate milk, hot chocolate, milkshakes or malts, regular soft drinks, fruit juices

Making Lasting Changes

Healthy eating is a cornerstone of good diabetes control. But changing your eating habits isn't always easy. To make those changes as painless as possible, you should plan to work closely with your dietitian or nutrition counselor to tailor your meal plan to your individual tastes and preferences. Sometimes you will have to make compromises between the kinds and amounts of food you prefer and what is best for your health. Your goal is to develop a meal plan that allows you to eat as many different foods as possible and to help keep the pleasure in eating.

Don't be too hard on yourself if you slip up now and then. Nobody's perfect. If you know ahead of time that you're going to find yourself in a situation in which you'll be tempted to stray from your usual eating—at a friend's wedding reception, for example—consider *beforehand* ways in which you can safely do so. You can scrape the icing off the cake, balance treats by reducing other foods, or exercise more later on.

CHAPTER 4

Exercising Control Over Your Diabetes

Generally speaking, there's no reason that you can't lead a full, physically active life when you have diabetes. In fact, there are plenty of good reasons that you *should* engage in regular physical activity. A regular exercise program can

- improve insulin sensitivity in your body. An active body burns sugar faster and more efficiently than an inactive one. During physical activity—even walking at a steady pace for half an hour—your muscles burn much more glucose than when your body is at rest.

- possibly reduce your need for diabetes medication. Since exercise increases insulin sensitivity, many people find that after several months of regular exercise, they can reduce the amount of insulin or oral medication they take.

- improve overall diabetes control. Moderate exercise has been shown to lower blood sugar levels among people with non-insulin-dependent diabetes, sometimes for several hours after they finish exercising. Because of this, regular exercise may, over time, lower overall blood sugar concentrations.

• help control your weight. Exercise burns calories and fat, and is as important as the foods you eat in controlling your weight. Overweight people who exercise while dieting are more successful in getting the weight off and keeping it off than those who lose weight by dieting alone. (Remember: if you are overweight and have non-insulin-dependent diabetes, losing weight is an essential part of diabetes control.)

• reduce your risk of cardiovascular disease. A sedentary lifestyle is now considered one of the major risk factors for heart disease. (Cigarette smoking, high blood pressure, and high blood cholesterol are the other major risk factors.) Exercise lowers your blood pressure and heart rate, allowing the heart to pump blood more efficiently. Regular physical activity also raises levels of high-density lipoprotein (HDL) cholesterol, the "good" cholesterol that guards against heart disease. Some studies have shown that exercise raises levels of plasminogen, an anticoagulant that may protect against the formation of blood clots in the arteries. (Blood clots can trigger a heart attack or stroke.) Scientists believe that these and possibly other effects of exercise on the body help protect physically active people from developing heart disease, one of the most prevalent and serious long-term complications associated with diabetes.

• help you feel better physically and emotionally. Exercise increases your energy level and boosts your self-esteem. Exercise is great for reducing tension and stress as well.

Adding exercise to your daily routine may be one of the easiest and most enjoyable changes you make in your lifestyle. Because you have diabetes, however, you will need to take a few extra precautions when exercising, particularly if you have insulin-dependent diabetes. These precautions are simple and easy to build into a fitness program.

First Things First: A Pre-exercise Review and Physical

Life is full of risks, and exercise is no exception. Even people without diabetes are subject to certain exercise-related risks, particularly overuse injuries, such as muscle strains and sprains. Because exercise affects the body's use of insulin, people with diabetes—particularly those taking insulin or oral medication—may be at a greater risk of developing low blood sugar while exercising and for several hours afterward. Here's what happens: When you exercise, your body must quickly mobilize energy reserves to fuel its working muscles with oxygen and nutrients. In people who don't have diabetes, this is a complex process in which insulin levels fall and other hormones rise, helping to release fat stored in your fat tissues and stepping up the liver's production of glucose. Normally, the liver produces precisely the amount of glucose needed by the exercising muscles, and blood glucose levels remain relatively stable. When you have diabetes, the effect of exercise on your blood sugar levels varies, depending on a number of factors, including how well your diabetes is controlled, your blood glucose levels when you start exercising, the intensity and duration of your workout, and your overall fitness level. The most important variable, however, is the level of insulin in your body during and after your exercise session. And while insulin levels fall in people who don't have diabetes, insulin levels in people with insulin-dependent diabetes sometimes rise because of the increased circulation in the area where the insulin was injected. This can result in episodes of hypoglycemia, since insulin helps the muscles absorb glucose from the bloodstream and slows the liver's production of glucose.

Some people who have had diabetes for years may have nerve and circulatory problems (including heart disease) that affect the type and level of exercise they can do. Most of these problems can be easily managed by taking a few extra precautions. You should start by having a complete physical examination and fitness evaluation before you begin exercising.

Your doctor will check your blood sugar levels to determine how well your diabetes is being controlled. You should also undergo a thorough cardiovascular examination, including a check of your blood pressure and blood cholesterol levels. If you are over forty, have a history of cardiovascular disease, or have had diabetes for more than fifteen years, an electrocardiogram (ECG or EKG) may be in order. This test measures your heart's rate and rhythm and its electrical activity while you are sitting still or lying down, and can detect possible signs of heart disease. You may also be advised to have an exercise stress test, which is an ECG performed while you exercise on a treadmill or stationary bicycle. An exercise stress test can be used to detect such problems as narrowing of the coronary arteries. It is also an ideal way to determine your level of cardiovascular fitness. An X ray picture of the chest may be made to evaluate the size and shape of the heart and the health of your lungs. Your doctor will also determine whether you have any nerve damage that would interfere with your ability to exercise; this will include an examination of your feet to check for possible nerve damage, which can result in *insensitive feet*. You should also have a complete eye examination to test your vision and determine whether you have a vision-threatening type of eye disease associated with diabetes, known as *diabetic retinopathy*.

If you have medical complications, such as poorly controlled blood sugar levels, high blood pressure, nerve damage, diabetic retinopathy, or an inability to detect signs of hypoglycemia *(hypoglycemic unawareness)*, you will need to be careful when you exercise, and you may have to be more discriminating about the types of exercise you choose. If you have cardiovascular disease, you should have an exercise program developed through a cardiac rehabilitation program. You may also be advised to exercise caution if you take large doses of aspirin, beta blockers, or other drugs that are known to cause hypoglycemia. (See page 72 for a more complete list.)

What Type of Exercise Is Best?

The best types of exercise for people with diabetes are aerobic activities, the kind that you do for an extended period to increase your heart rate and breathing. Aerobic exercises, such as walking, bicycling, swimming, and jogging, strengthen your heart, lungs, and circulatory system, and help improve insulin sensitivity.

Brisk walking is one of the best exercises for beginners because it requires no special skills or equipment, and you can walk practically anywhere. Bicycling and swimming are good, enjoyable low-impact activities, too. Jogging and running give you an excellent aerobic workout, but the risk of suffering an injury is somewhat greater than that for walking. You'll also need special footwear designed to help absorb some of the shock of this high-impact activity. (Note: If you plan to jog or run, you should have a careful evaluation of your feet by a qualified health care professional; be sure to ask your doctor or diabetes educator about selecting proper footwear.)

Aerobic dancing, hiking, and team sports are not as highly recommended, since you may not have as much control over your level of activity in these sports, and it's easy to overextend yourself. The risk of suffering an exercise-related injury, such as a muscle sprain or strain, is also greater with these activities.

Weight lifting or other stationary exercises are good for strengthening your muscles, but these activities do little to strengthen your heart muscle or improve insulin sensitivity. If you lift weights, be sure to participate in some kind of aerobic activity as well.

Certain medical complications may influence your choice of activities:

If you have insensitive feet: Avoid running and jogging, as well as team sports and other activities that involve running. Running can injure your feet without your being aware of it. Better activities for you are bicycling and swimming.

If you have diabetic retinopathy: Avoid strenuous, high-intensity exercises, such as weight lifting and isometric exercises for the upper body. These exercises can raise your blood pressure and put undue strain on the delicate blood vessels in your eyes, possibly causing them to break and bleed. You should also avoid activities that require your head to be lower than your midsection more than briefly, such as certain yoga positions. This could increase the pressure on the blood vessels in your eyes.

If you have hypertension: Avoid heavy lifting or straining, which can raise your blood pressure. You should also avoid intense exercises involving the arms and upper body, such as push-ups and pull-ups. Upper-body exercises cause greater increases in blood pressure than activities involving the legs and lower-body muscles. Rhythmic exercises involving the legs, such as walking, jogging, and cycling, are better choices.

How Much Exercise Do You Need?

To get the most benefit from aerobic exercise, you must raise your heart rate to a working level and keep it there for at least twenty minutes. For most people, this means exercising strenuously enough to raise your heart rate to between 60 and 80 percent of its maximum capacity, what's known as your *target heart range*. If you haven't had an exercise stress test, you can calculate your target heart range using the equation here:

220 − your age × .60 to .80 = your target heart range

Here's an example for a forty-five-year-old man or woman:

220 − 45 = 175 × .60 to .80 = 105 to 140

So if you are forty-five years old, your target heart range is 105 to 140 beats per minute.

To ensure that you are exercising within your target heart range, you should monitor your heart rate while you exercise. This involves periodically taking your pulse at either the carotid artery in your neck or the radial artery in your wrist (see illustration). To measure your carotid pulse, place the index and middle finger of your right hand on the left side of your throat. To measure your radial pulse, place the two fingers of your right hand on your left wrist, below the thumb. Now, using a digital watch that shows seconds or a clock with a second hand, count your pulse for ten seconds and multiply the number of pulse beats by six. Your pulse beats should fall somewhere within your target range.

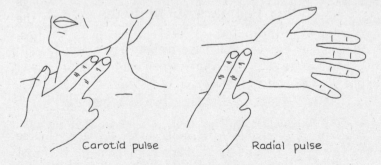

Carotid pulse   Radial pulse

How to Take Your Pulse

Most experts recommend that you exercise at this level three to four times per week until you become more physically fit. (Your doctor can help you set appropriate fitness goals.) You can usually stay fit by exercising at least three times a week thereafter.

Each exercise session should include a warm-up and cooldown period. Start each exercise session with five to ten minutes of stretching exercises and moderate aerobic activity. This increases the blood flow to your heart and muscles, preparing your body for more strenuous activity. After the aerobic portion of your workout, you should spend the next fifteen to twenty minutes cooling down with less strenuous exercise, such as walking and stretches. A cool-down period is particularly important for several reasons. When you stop exercising abruptly, the extra blood diverted to your muscles during the exercise may pool in your legs, causing a dangerous shortage of blood to either your brain or your heart. This could make you feel dizzy or even pass out. A cool-down period also helps prevent the buildup of lactic acid in your muscles, a major cause of postexercise muscle soreness.

Some Safety Guidelines for People with Diabetes

Remember: because you have diabetes, you will have to take some extra safety measures when exercising to prevent hypoglycemia or hyperglycemia.

• Carry a wallet card or wear a bracelet that says you have diabetes.

• Bring along a high-carbohydrate drink or snack, such as orange juice, glucose tablets or gel, or hard candy, to prevent or treat hypoglycemia during or after exercise. This is especially important if you take insulin or oral medication.

• Be alert for signs and symptoms of hypoglycemia while you are exercising and for several hours afterward. Early signs include excessive hunger, sweating, shakiness, or heart palpitations. Obviously, exercise itself can cause you to break out in a sweat and cause your heart to beat faster. You may have to periodically stop exercising and test your blood sugar. Make sure your exercise partner knows the signs and symptoms of hypoglycemia and, if you take insulin, knows how to give a glucagon injection. (See page 108 for instructions.)

• Drink plenty of sugar-free fluids, such as water or diet soda, before, during, and after your workout to avoid dehydration. On particularly hot days, you may want to exercise in an air-conditioned building or skip exercising altogether.

• Periodically monitor your blood sugar levels before, during, and after exercising (see Chapter 6) to see how your body responds to exercise. If you take insulin or oral medication, you and your physician can use this information to make appropriate adjustments in your insulin dosage and calorie intake.

As a general rule, you won't need to adjust your insulin dosage if you exercise moderately for less than thirty to forty-five minutes, but you will probably need to eat a high-protein, high-carbohydrate snack, such as a granola bar, just before your workout. Your doctor or nutrition counselor will help you determine the size of the snack.

If you experience hypoglycemia several hours after exercising, you may be advised to eat a small snack just after your workout. If you exercise in the evening, you will be instructed to monitor your blood sugar levels and adjust your nighttime snack to ensure that you don't experience hypoglycemia during the night.

If you exercise strenuously for more than forty-five minutes, your doctor may recommend a reduction in your insulin dosage. You should also avoid injecting insulin in the arm or leg that will be predominantly used for exercise, since the massaging action of the working muscles and the increased circulation could increase the rate of insulin absorption.

• Avoid drinking alcoholic beverages just before or after exercising. Alcohol can increase your risk of developing hypoglycemia *and* can contribute to dehydration.

• If you experience extreme discomfort or pain (other than normal muscle strain), severe shortness of breath, lightheadedness, or nausea, stop exercising immediately, take some carbohydrate, and call your doctor if the symptoms don't pass quickly.

• Work with your doctor to make appropriate adjustments in the amount of insulin you take on the days you plan to exercise.

Keeping Your Interest Level High

Once you've received your doctor's approval to start exercising and have chosen an appropriate activity, you're ready to begin. To increase your odds of successfully starting and sticking with an exercise program, try these tips:

Choose an activity that you enjoy and that is convenient for you. If you decide that swimming would be a good exercise for you, but don't have ready access to a swimming pool, you're not likely to exercise as often as you should. Again, brisk walking is an ideal activity because it requires no spe-

cial skills or equipment and you can walk practically anywhere.

Make a contract with yourself—and with your physician—to exercise regularly. Often, making a commitment
in writing helps to keep you motivated. State your exercise
goals in the contract, too, as well as a time frame for meeting those goals. When you've reached those goals, set new
ones.

Start slowly. If you have been sedentary for a while, start
with short (five to ten minutes), frequent (five to seven days
per week) sessions. This helps to gradually condition your
body for more strenuous activity and to make exercise an integral part of your day. Gradually work your way up to
longer, more strenuous exercise sessions.

Exercise every day, if you can. Although three to four days
of strenuous activity is all that's needed to increase cardiovascular fitness, you're much more likely to keep the habit of
exercising if you do it daily. In addition, the effects of exercise on your blood sugar levels are short-lived, lasting only a
few days. Hypoglycemia is particularly risky for people who
exercise sporadically while continuing to take their usual insulin dose. So by exercising every day—if possible, around
the same time every day—you may help head off hypoglycemic episodes.

Vary your routine. If you get tired of the same old exercise
routine, change it. Instead of walking one day, ride your bicycle. Or choose a different route to walk.

Exercise with a partner. You won't feel so alone or bored.
A partner can provide encouragement and support on the
days you don't feel like exercising. You can do the same for
your partner at times, too.

Reward yourself. After you've reached one or more of your
exercise goals, do more than give yourself a pat on the back.
Treat yourself to a new pair of exercise shoes, a movie, or an
item of clothing you've had your eye on.

Whatever you do, keep in mind that almost any activity is better than none at all. Even small increases in your normal daily activities, such as walking to the store instead of driving, or taking the stairs instead of the elevator, can help.

CHAPTER 5

Diabetes Medications

If you have non-insulin-dependent diabetes and can't control it through diet and exercise alone, or if your blood sugar levels at the time you are diagnosed are exceptionally high, your doctor may prescribe medications that lower blood glucose concentrations. These include a class of drugs known as *oral hypoglycemic agents*, taken in the form of a pill, or insulin shots. Of course, insulin will be prescribed for *all* people with insulin-dependent diabetes.

Oral Hypoglycemic Medications

These drugs, also known as *sulfonylureas*, are *not* "insulin pills." In fact, in order for the drugs to work, your body must produce *some* insulin, so they're not helpful for people with insulin-dependent diabetes.

It's not known exactly how these drugs work. When you first start taking oral hypoglycemic medications, they *in-*

crease insulin secretion by the pancreas so that there is enough insulin to clear excess sugar from the bloodstream. After several months of therapy, however, insulin levels fall back to pretreatment levels, yet blood sugar levels may remain stable. Experts believe the drugs continue working for several reasons: The medications reduce the rate at which the liver releases glucose into the bloodstream, keeping blood glucose concentrations low. Oral medications may also overcome insulin resistance by increasing the number of insulin receptors on your body's cells and by somehow improving the cells' ability to process glucose.

Some people respond better to oral hypoglycemic medications than others. You may be a good candidate for these drugs if you

- developed diabetes after the age of forty
- have had diabetes for less than five years
- are of normal weight or overweight
- have never taken insulin or have taken less than 40 units per day

Oral hypoglycemic agents aren't for everybody, however. As mentioned earlier, people with insulin-dependent diabetes aren't helped by oral hypoglycemic medications, since their bodies produce virtually no insulin. In addition, scientists still don't know what effect the drugs might have on a developing fetus or breast-feeding infant. So if you are pregnant or nursing a baby, oral drugs are not an option. Similarly, even if you do well with these drugs, they may not be effective when you have a serious medical condition, such as an infection. They cannot be used if you are allergic to such medications (sulfa drugs).

When deciding whether you should use oral medications or insulin therapy, your physician will consider:

1. how high your blood sugar level is at the time of diagnosis
2. your age and weight

3. your motivation (treating yourself with an insulin injection takes a bit more initiative than taking a pill)

4. your personal preference, once you have a complete picture of what to expect from either treatment

There are several kinds of oral hypoglycemic agents, which differ in their potency and in the way they are processed in your body. Your physician can help you determine which form of the drug is best suited to your needs. Here's a look at what is available to you:

Tolbutamide (brand name *Orinase;* also available by its generic name) is the least potent of the sulfonylureas and is considered by some the safest. (Tolbutamide can even be taken by people with kidney problems.) Effects of the drug last from six to twelve hours, so it must be taken two to three times per day.

Chlorpropamide (brand name *Diabinese;* also available by its generic name) is one of the most potent oral hypoglycemic agents. The drug's effects last up to sixty hours, so it is taken only once a day. Side effects include water retention and abnormal lowering of sodium levels in the blood.

Tolazamide (brand name *Tolinase;* also available by its generic name) lasts from twelve to twenty-four hours and is taken once or twice a day.

Acetazolamide (brand name *Dymelor*) is taken once or twice a day and lasts from twelve to eighteen hours. The drug acts as a diuretic, and causes increased excretion of uric acid in the urine. The drug is not widely prescribed today.

Glipizide (brand name *Glucotrol)* is one of the newer "second-generation" sulfonylureas. The drug remains active in your body from twelve to twenty-four hours, and may be taken once or twice a day. It is as effective as chlorpropamide in lowering blood sugar levels and has fewer side effects.

Glyburide (brand names *Diabeta* and *Micronase)* is another "second-generation" sulfonylurea, lasting from sixteen to twenty-four hours in the bloodstream. This drug may be taken once or twice a day. Again, the drug is as effective as chlorpropamide in lowering blood sugar levels, but with fewer side effects.

One of the most serious side effects associated with *all* oral hypoglycemic agents is severe hypoglycemia. People who take chlorpropamide, in particular, are prone to episodes of hypoglycemia because of the length of time the drug remains active in the body. Elderly people who take oral hypoglycemic drugs are also more susceptible to hypoglycemia, especially those who tend to skip meals and those who have liver, kidney, or cardiovascular problems.

If you are at a greater risk of suffering hypoglycemic episodes, your physician may prescribe one of the less potent drugs. If you experience symptoms of hypoglycemia (shakiness, sweating, fatigue, hunger, a rapid heartbeat, irritability, or confusion) while taking any of these drugs, follow the instructions for coping with hypoglycemia in Chapter 7, "Emergencies." You should notify your doctor as well; he or she may want to adjust your dosage or have you switch to another oral medication.

Other uncommon side effects include adverse blood reactions, such as anemia (an abnormal drop in the number of red blood cells or platelets), skin reactions (rashes, reddish or purplish spots, or itching), thyroid problems, or heart problems. Some people develop digestive problems, such as nausea, vomiting, or *cholestasis*, an interruption of bile flow from the liver, which results in large pale stools, itching and possibly jaundice. These problems resolve once you stop taking the drugs. If you experience any of these side effects while taking oral hypoglycemic medications, your doctor may recommend that you change to insulin.

If you take oral medication, you should be aware that many other medications may interact with these drugs, either exacerbating or interfering with their ability to lower blood sugar. (You'll find some of the most important drugs listed in the table that follows.) For this reason, people who take oral hypoglycemic agents should be carefully monitored by a physician while taking other medications. *Always* call your doctor before you take *any* other medication—even such a seemingly safe over-the-counter drug as ibuprofen (Advil, Motrin).

Once you and your physician have decided on a medication, you will be given the lowest effective dose. The dosage will then be increased every one or two weeks until your blood sugar drops to safer levels or until you are taking the maximum dose of the drug. If the drug doesn't adequately control your diabetes, your doctor may have you change to another oral medication. (Two oral hypoglycemic drugs *don't* work better than one, so your doctor won't prescribe more than one at a time.) If the new drug doesn't control your blood sugar levels, you may have to take insulin.

Between 60 and 70 percent of the people who try oral hypoglycemic agents are able to effectively control their glucose levels. Keep in mind, however, that oral medications are an *adjunct* to improved eating and regular exercise, not a substitute for them. You will still have to follow your prescribed eating plan (and exercise regularly) when taking these drugs.

Sometimes oral hypoglycemic drugs effectively control blood sugar levels for a while, then stop working. This occurs most commonly among people who do not continue to follow their eating plan. The drugs often start working again once they return to healthier eating habits. Oral medications may also stop working if you have an underlying disease or condition that affects blood sugar levels, such as an infection, pregnancy, or cardiovascular disease. If this is the case, you may have to temporarily change to insulin shots until the condition is treated (or, in the case of pregnancy, until after the baby is born). If the drugs cease to control your blood sugar levels because your diabetes has worsened, you may have to permanently take insulin shots.

Medications that May Cause Drug Interactions with Oral Hypoglycemic Agents

The following common prescription drugs may interact with oral diabetes medications, causing a greater than expected drop in blood sugar levels or interfering with your diabetes medication's ability to lower blood sugar. This is just a sampling of the most commonly prescribed drugs, so check with your doctor or pharmacist before taking *any* other medication (prescription or over-the-counter) along with your diabetes pills.

Drugs that May Cause Hypoglycemia

Generic Name or class of drug	Brand Name	Commonly Prescribed for
Beta blockers	Biocadren, Brevibloc, Cartrol, Corgard, Corzide, Inderal, Inderide, Kerlone, Levatol, Lopressor, Normozide, Sectral, Tenoretic, Timolide, Visken	Hypertension, heart disease
Clofibrate	Atromid	Hyperlipidemia (high cholesterol or triglycerides)
Guanethidine	Esimil, Ismelin	Hypertension
Monoamine oxidase inhibitors	Nardil, Parnate	Depression
Phenylbutazone	Butazolidin	Rheumatoid arthritis, gouty arthritis

Drugs that May Cause Hyperglycemia

Generic name or class of drug	*Brand Name*	*Commonly Prescribed for*
Beta blockers	Biocadren, Brevibloc, Cartrol, Corgard, Corzide, Inderal, Inderide, Kerlone, Levatol, Lopressor, Normozide, Sectral, Tenoretic, Timolide, Visken	Hypertension, heart disease
Diuretics (thiazides, furosemide)	Aldactazide, Aquatensen, Capozide, Corzide, Diucardin, Diuril, Diutensen, Dyazide, Enduron, Enduronyl, Esidrix, Exna, HydroDIURIL, Lasix, Maxzide, Minizide, Moduretic, Naturetin, Oretic, Oreticyl, Prinzide, Rauzide, Renese, Saluron, Vaseretic, Zestoretic,	Hypertension
Estrogens	Emcyt; Estrace; Estraderm; Premarin; Estratest; Menrium; Ogen; Brevicon; Demulen; Estinyl; Levlen; Lo/Ovral; Loestrin; Modicon; Nelova; Nordette; Norethin; Norinyl;	Postmenopausal hormone therapy, oral contraception

	Norlestrin; Ortho-Novum 1/35, 7-7-7, 10/11; Ovcon; Ovral; Tri-Levlen; Tri-Norinyl; Triphasil	
Indomethacin	Indocin	Arthritis pain
Nicotinic acid	Niacin, Niacor, Nicobid, Nicolar, Slo-Niacin	High cholesterol
Phenytoin	Dilantin	Epilepsy, seizures

Aspirin and aspirin-containing products also tend to lower blood sugar levels and should be used with caution by people taking oral hypoglycemic medications. And as mentioned on page 42, alcohol is a potent hypoglycemic agent, particularly when you drink on an empty stomach. If you take oral hypoglycemic medications, you should exercise extreme caution when you drink alcoholic beverages. If you drink at all, make sure you eat something first.

Insulin Therapy

If you have insulin-dependent diabetes, you must take insulin to live, and you will have to take insulin for the rest of your life. But even if you have non-insulin-dependent diabetes, you may have to take insulin from time to time, such as when you suffer an injury or illness, when you are pregnant, or when you have surgery. Some people with non-insulin-dependent diabetes must take insulin regularly. Indeed, many physicians prefer insulin over oral medications for people with non-insulin-dependent diabetes that is not improved by weight control alone.

Insulin shots reduce blood sugar levels in the same way as insulin produced by the pancreas: by helping your body's tissues absorb glucose, and by suppressing the production of glucose by the liver. Insulin also helps your body's liver, muscle, and fat tissues absorb triglycerides (fats circulating in the bloodstream).

The good news: in the past ten years, vast improvements have been made in the types of insulin available to you and in the way insulin is delivered into your body. So taking insulin is easier now than ever before.

Insulin therapy must be individualized for each patient, so you should work with your doctor to decide which insulin and insulin delivery system is best for you. Start by familiarizing yourself with the various insulins and insulin delivery products available.

Insulins

When insulin was first discovered in 1922, only one type— rapid-acting insulin (called Regular insulin in the United States)—was available to people with diabetes. What's more, all insulin came from pig or cow pancreases, and its purity and strength were not always reliable. Today, there are more than forty insulins to choose from, including genetically manufactured "human" insulin.

When deciding which insulin is best for you, you and your doctor will want to consider the *type* of insulin you take (for instance, whether the insulin is short-acting or long-acting), and the *source* of the insulin. These factors affect the drug's *onset* (its rate of absorption by the body), its *peak time* (the time during which the insulin is at its maximum strength in terms of lowering blood glucose), and its *duration* (the period during which the insulin continues to lower blood sugar).

Types of Insulin

The type of insulin you take is defined by how soon it starts to lower glucose levels after it has been injected, and how long it lasts. (Keep in mind that each person responds differently to insulin, so the times here are estimates.) All insulin bottles are labeled with a letter to indicate which type of insulin is inside.

Regular or *short-acting insulin*, labeled with a capital "R," enters the bloodstream approximately thirty minutes after injection. It peaks one and a half to three hours after injection, and remains active in the bloodstream about five to seven hours.

Semilente, labeled with a capital "S," is a special type of short-acting insulin that takes effect one to two hours after injection. It reaches its peak three to eight hours later and continues working for ten to sixteen hours.

Buffered Regular insulin, also labeled "R," is a short-acting insulin specially made for use with insulin pumps. (For more on insulin pumps, see "Insulin Delivery Systems," which follows.)

Intermediate-acting insulin reaches the bloodstream about two to four hours after injection. It peaks four to fourteen hours later and stays in the bloodstream about eighteen to twenty-four hours. Two common types of intermediate-acting insulin are *NPH* (labeled "N") and *Lente* (labeled "L"). The recently introduced human Ultralente, labeled "U," is considered a long-acting insulin, but because people absorb insulin at different rates, it may be used as an intermediate-acting insulin for some people.

Long-acting insulins usually don't peak until fourteen to twenty-four hours after injection and remain active in the bloodstream for twenty to thirty-six hours, providing a nearly continuous insulin release. Long-acting insulins include *Ultralente* and *human Ultralente* (both labeled "U").

Premixed insulins are a combination of short- and intermediate-acting insulins. The only currently available mixture is 70 percent NPH insulin and 30 percent Regular insulin. The Regular insulin starts acting within approximately 30 minutes after injection, and the NPH takes over after the Regular insulin has peaked. The mixture is labeled "70/30."

Your physician may recommend that you take more than one kind of insulin in a twenty-four-hour period to help balance your changing need for insulin throughout the day. For example, if your doctor prescribes a long- or intermediate-acting insulin to help your body maintain a constant glucose level, he or she may also prescribe a short-acting insulin to be taken at mealtimes when glucose levels jump. You may be instructed to mix two types of insulin in a syringe for one injection, or you may be given a prescription for a premixed solution.

Sources of Insulin

The nonhuman sources of insulin are *beef pancreas* and *pork pancreas*. The beef and pork insulins are often mixed. In the past, impurities in animal insulin preparations were associated with a greater risk of such side effects as allergic reactions and the formation of antibodies to insulin that could compromise the drug's ability to lower blood sugar levels. Thanks to dramatic advances in the purification of these products, however, highly purified animal insulins today contain less than 10 parts per million of impurities, reducing the likelihood of side effects. Pure pork insulin is the purest of the animal insulins, but it is also more expensive than beef or beef-pork insulin.

More and more people with diabetes today are taking the recently developed *human insulin*. "Human" insulin is a bit of a misnomer, since it *does not* come from human beings. *Semisynthetic human insulin* is made by changing pork insulin through a chemical process into a form identical to human insulin; *recombinant insulin* is made through genetic technology. Both of these insulins are chemically identical to the insulin made by the human body.

Human insulin is preferred by many physicians because it is considered purer than animal insulins (it contains less than one part per million of impurities) and hence is less likely to trigger an allergic reaction. In addition, human insulin is less likely to trigger the formation of *antibodies* by your body's immune defense system, which could neutralize the blood-sugar-lowering effects of insulin. (Some researchers believe that antibodies may actually bind with the insulin and release it into the bloodstream later, resulting in unpredictable levels of insulin in the bloodstream.) If you use human insulin, you should be aware that it acts faster, peaks earlier, and has a shorter duration of effect than animal insulins.

In the future, human insulin may replace all other currently available types of insulin. If you are already using an animal insulin and don't have any allergic problems, however, there's no need to switch to a human insulin.

Insulin Strengths

In the United States, the only generally available strength or *concentration* of insulin is 100 units of insulin per milliliter of fluid, or *U-100*. U-100 insulin bottles are sold with orange caps. In Europe and Latin America, insulin is also available as U-40, or 40 units of insulin per milliliter of liquid. Some bottles of U-40 insulin are also sold in the United States; they have red caps.

Knowing the amount of insulin in each milliliter or cc of liquid matters, as you must match the concentration of the insulin with the appropriate syringe. (U-100 syringes, which have orange tops, match a U-100 solution; likewise U-40 syringes, which have red tops, match a U-40 solution.) While a mismatch is unlikely to occur, you should be aware of this difference if you travel. *If you draw up a U-100 solution in a U-40 syringe, you'll draw up two and a half times the amount of insulin you need.* (For more travel tips, see page 162.)

Insulin Delivery Systems

Once you and your physician have decided on the best type of insulin for you, you'll need a way to deliver it into your body. There's no shortage of options.

All but a few people use syringes, which are smaller and more portable than they used to be. Also, the needles are smaller and have sharp points and special coatings to make the injection as easy and painless as possible. Most people find that when injections are given properly (see "Preparing and Giving an Insulin Injection," which follows), they are almost painless.

You may want to try several different brands of syringes before deciding on the one that is most comfortable for you. When shopping, make sure the syringe is the *right size* for your dosage. If you are taking 45-unit doses, you can't use a 30-unit syringe. You may also want to check the syringe barrel to make sure you can easily read the markings. Some syringes have a plunger that's a different color to make it easier for you to draw up your dosage.

If you feel squeamish about injecting yourself, you might want to try an insulin *insertion aid*. These are spring-loaded devices that usually hide the needle. After positioning the device over the injection site, you simply press a button, move a lever, or press down on the device to release the spring, which automatically inserts the needle into the skin. Ask your physician about these devices. He or she might have one you could try.

If you must take multiple injections during the day, there are several alternatives to syringes, including insulin *infusers*, *pens*, *jets*, and *pumps*. Insulin *infusers* create a portal through which you can inject insulin, minimizing needle punctures. A plastic tube is inserted into the fatty tissue just under the skin and remains taped in place for forty-eight to seventy-two hours. You then use a syringe to inject the insulin through the plastic tube. Some people are prone to developing infections with infusers.

An insulin *pen* is like an old-fashioned cartridge pen, but instead of a penpoint, it has a needle, and instead of an ink cartridge, it has an insulin cartridge. These devices are particularly handy for people who take multiple injections and whose coordination is impaired.

Another device for delivering insulin into your body is called a *jet injector.* Jet injectors do not actually pierce the skin; rather, they use pressure to send a stream of insulin through the skin. Some people have problems with bruising and insulin absorption rates with these devices. Ask your physician for more information on these devices.

Insulin pumps are tiny computerized pumps, about the size of a call-beeper, that you wear in your pocket or on a belt. The pump delivers a regulated amount of insulin through a plastic tube and a small needle that is inserted under the fatty layer of your skin (usually on your stomach). The needle and tube remain taped in place. (With the Sof-set tube, only the tube stays under your skin.)

If you use an insulin pump, you must monitor your glucose levels at least four time a day (see Chapter 6) and learn how to make adjustments in your insulin, food, and exercise in response to the test results. You will initially spend a great deal of time with your health care team determining just how much insulin you need at different times of the day. Because of the large amount of glucose testing required and the difficulties of establishing an insulin injection schedule, pumps are not for everyone. Some people may find it awkward to wear the pump twenty-four hours a day.

When considering any of these devices, be sure to check with your insurance company to see what it will cover. Shop around for prices, too. Before you decide on an alternative method of injection, be sure to discuss with your health care team the benefits and potential problems you might encounter.

You may also want to get a copy of the *Buyer's Guide to Diabetes Products* published annually by the American Diabetes

Association (see page 187 for the address), which has a list of all currently available insulins and insulin delivery products.

How Much Insulin Will You Need?

The amount of insulin you take every day varies according to your weight, body build (the ratio of fat to muscle), level of physical activity, daily food intake, other medications, general health, daily stress level, and the type of diabetes you have. People with non-insulin-dependent diabetes may need as little as 5 to 10 units of insulin per day. If you have had diabetes for many years, however, are overweight, or have moderate to severe hyperglycemia, you are probably more resistant to insulin and may require large doses of insulin— possibly 100 or more units per day—to regulate your blood sugar levels. Moreover, your need for insulin will likely increase over time as your cells become increasingly insulin-resistant. Indeed, the insulin required to control glucose levels among people with non-insulin-dependent diabetes can increase as much as five-fold over a ten-year period.

If you have non-insulin-dependent diabetes and take less than 30 units of insulin per day, you may be able to get by with only one injection of an intermediate-acting insulin just before breakfast. If you take more than 30 units per day, you will probably need to take a mixture of Regular and intermediate-acting insulin, once before breakfast and again before supper. If you are particularly resistant to insulin, your physician may recommend a combination of oral therapy and two injections of a mix of Regular and intermediate-acting insulin per day.

If you have insulin-dependent diabetes, you won't necessarily need *more* insulin than a person with non-insulin-dependent diabetes, but you will probably have to take at least two injections per day; one injection in the morning usually will not provide you with the glucose control you need to last until after supper and into the night. A dose of intermediate-acting insulin, alone or with added regular insulin, before breakfast and supper may be sufficient to carry you through both the day and night. If two injections fail to keep your glucose under control, you may have to take a third injection before lunch or just before bedtime.

MDI (multidose insulin) therapy is another alternative. A person on an MDI therapy plan might take three injections of short-acting insulin at mealtimes, and a longer-acting preparation at night. The goal is to mimic the patterns of insulin secretion that you would have if you didn't have diabetes. Therefore, shots are given at meals, when glucose typically rises and when the body would secrete higher levels of insulin.

For people who wish to achieve strict diabetes control, an insulin pump may be in order. Insulin pumps are computer-operated and inject a continuous stream of short-acting insulin into your blood. At mealtimes, you can give yourself an insulin burst to counteract rising glucose levels. Called *continuous subcutaneous insulin infusion* (CSII), this form of therapy, like MDI, is used as an intensive treatment to help normalize blood glucose levels. In studies, neither MDI nor an insulin pump is superior in attaining control.

Both MDI and CSII therapies require a large commitment from both you and your health care team. You will have to monitor your glucose levels at least four times a day and keep careful written records, and you will require more visits to your doctor than people who take fewer injections.

Many people with newly diagnosed insulin-dependent diabetes, particularly adolescents and adults, start producing insulin again within weeks after beginning insulin therapy. This is known as the *honeymoon phase* of insulin-dependent diabetes and may last for several weeks or months. During this time, you will have to reduce your insulin dosage accordingly. Eventually, however—usually within six to eighteen months of beginning insulin therapy—your insulin needs will increase again.

Side Effects of Insulin Therapy

Anyone who takes insulin risks suffering occasional episodes of low blood sugar, or hypoglycemia. You should familiarize yourself with the symptoms and treatment of low blood sugar so that you will know what to do if it happens to you. (You'll find complete instructions for coping with a hypoglycemic episode in Chapter 7, "Emergencies.") If you take insulin, you should also keep a glucagon emergency kit on hand and *make sure that family, friends, coworkers, and exercise partners know how to give a glucagon injection.* (See Chapter 7.) Glucagon, a drug that raises blood sugar, must be administered when your blood sugar levels fall so low that you pass out.

Other side effects include allergic reactions, insulin resistance, and *lipodystrophies* (either a loss of or excess accumulation of fat tissue at the injection site).

Allergic reactions: Some people, particularly those using the less pure beef or beef-pork insulins, may experience skin reactions at the injection site, usually within a month of beginning insulin therapy. Red, itchy spots will appear three to six hours *after* an injection and may persist for several days. (Some people experience a burning or stinging sensation at the time of the injection, followed by the formation of itchy, red welts several hours later.) Skin reactions to intermediate-acting insulins are more common than those to short-acting insulins and may be due to the carrier protein (protamine) in NPH insulin, or the zinc in Lente insulins.

If symptoms aren't too bothersome, your physician may recommend that you simply wait them out; most skin reactions clear up by themselves within several months. Sometimes switching to a zinc-free insulin helps. Your physician may also recommend small doses of injectable steroids (such as hydrocortisone) or antihistamines (such as Benadryl), which can be added to your insulin in the same syringe. Switching to pure pork or human insulin, or from one brand or type of insulin to another, may also help.

A generalized allergic reaction to insulin is very rare with modern insulins. It is more likely in people who stop taking insulin, then start taking it again, than in those who take insulin continuously. Symptoms include itchy, red hives that develop within thirty to sixty minutes of an injection and spread to a larger area surrounding the injection site. In some people, the allergic reaction spreads throughout the body.

If you suffer an allergic reaction, you will probably have to undergo desensitization, in which your normal insulin dose is cut back dramatically, followed by injections of very small amounts of insulin that are gradually increased over a matter of days. Your physician may also prescribe antihistamines and recommend that you switch to pure pork or human insulin.

Lipodystrophies: Some people may experience a loss of fat tissue at the site of insulin injections; this is known as *insulin-induced lipoatrophy.* The problem is most common in adolescent girls and young women, and while it is not medically a cause for concern, it can be a cosmetic problem, with hollowed-out areas or pits in the skin surface. Lipoatrophy is less common now that purification of insulins has improved. Ironically, one of the most effective treatments is to inject pure insulin preparations directly into the affected areas.

A related problem is an increase in the amount of fatty tissue at the injection site, known as *lipohypertrophy* or puffy areas caused by increased fat under the skin. This is more likely to occur if you repeatedly inject your insulin in the same place. If you develop areas of lipohypertrophy, you should avoid injecting your insulin in these areas, since absorption of insulin from these sites may be delayed and erratic. Another reason to change your injection site is that the extra tissue gradually disappears if you completely avoid injection into this site.

Another side effect of potential importance to people with non-insulin-dependent diabetes is increased appetite. This could trigger a vicious cycle of eating more, gaining weight, becoming more insulin-resistant, experiencing a rise in blood sugar levels, and requiring even more insulin. If you have non-insulin-dependent diabetes and take insulin, you will have to be extra careful with the foods you eat to avoid falling into this trap.

Insulin Therapy: A User's Guide

Once you and your physician have decided on the type and amount of insulin you need, you'll need to know how to purchase, store, and use it. Here are a few guidelines to follow.

Buying and Storing Insulin

Before purchasing your first bottle of insulin, you may want to shop around to find the cheapest, most convenient pharmacy. Prices of insulin can vary by several dollars per bottle. Sometimes you can buy insulin more cheaply if you buy in volume, so ask your pharmacist. You may also want to check with your insurance company to find out whether you are restricted to certain pharmacies. (Some insurance companies contract with specific pharmacies for lower prices and offer their customers lower prices *only* at those pharmacies.) Some pharmacies deliver, which could be crucial if you are too sick or too busy to pick up your insulin yourself.

Consider the pharmacist, too. Try to find a pharmacist who is familiar with diabetes testing and treatment products, who will take an interest in your medical problems, and who will alert you to any difficulties you might have with other medications.

When you buy insulin, you will need to know the *source* or *species* (human, beef, pork, or mixed beef-pork), the *brand name* (Humulin, Novolin, Iletin I, Iletin II, etc.), and the *kind* (NPH, Regular, Lente, etc.). In the United States, pharmacies will always provide U-100 insulin and syringes. Never change the species or type(s) of your insulin unless you first discuss the changes with your physician. Any alterations in insulin must be carefully monitored, as a new mix of types or change of species may require a change in dosage.

When you receive your insulin, check the species, brand name, and type against what you requested. Next check the expiration date. You must be able to use the entire bottle before this time. To determine whether or not you will have enough time to use the insulin, divide the number of units in the bottle by the number of units you take each day. For example, if you buy a 1,000-unit bottle of U-100 and use 35 units of insulin per day, divide 1,000 by 35:

1,000 units U-100 ÷ 35 units per day = 28 days of insulin

Next, check the insulin's appearance. Regular and Buffered Regular insulins should be clear and have *no* color. *Do not use* them if they look cloudy or thickened or have solid particles in them. All other insulins should look evenly *cloudy* (like skim milk) after you gently mix them by rolling the bottle between the palms of your hands. *Do not use* these insulin preparations if, after mixing them, there is insulin on the bottom, there are clumps of insulin in the liquid, or there are solid pieces of insulin sticking to the bottom or sides of the bottle. (Your bottle will have a slightly "frosted" look on the inside if the insulin is sticking.) If your insulin doesn't look as it should, take it back to the pharmacy for a refund or exchange.

After buying your insulin, be sure to store it correctly. The manufacturers recommend storing it in the refrigerator, but cold insulin makes for a more painful injection. This can be resolved by drawing up the insulin and letting it sit for a few minutes to come to room temperature. Never put your insulin in direct sunlight or in the freezer. Always check the expiration date and for clarity or cloudiness of the liquid again just before using it.

Preparing and Giving an Insulin Injection

Your doctor or an assistant will teach you how to prepare and inject your insulin. Use the steps here as a reminder once you begin doing it on your own.

Preparing a Single Dose of Insulin

1. Wash your hands.
2. Mix your insulin by rolling the bottle gently between your palms, turning the bottle end over end a few times, or agitating the bottle gently.
3. If this is a new bottle of insulin, remove the colored cap, leaving the rubber stopper and metal band in place.
4. Clean the rubber stopper with an alcohol swab. (This step is not necessary if you are using a newly uncapped bottle.)
5. Take the cover off the needle. Pull back the plunger until the tip of the plunger is at the number of units you intend to take. Your syringe is now full of air.
6. Push the needle through the rubber stopper. Press in the plunger to push the air into the bottle of insulin.
7. Turn the bottle and syringe upside down with the tip of the needle in the insulin. Hold the bottle with one hand and pull back on the plunger with the other hand. This pulls insulin into the syringe. Pull the plunger back slowly until the tip of the plunger is even with your dosage amount.
8. *Before* you take the needle out of the rubber stopper, look at the insulin in the syringe. If you see air bubbles, slowly push the plunger down to put the insulin back in the bottle, then slowly pull the syringe out again. Repeat this until there are no large air bubbles in the syringe.
9. Double-check your dosage.
10. Pull the needle out of the rubber stopper. If you need to lay down the syringe before giving yourself the in-

jection, put the cap back on the needle. Now you are
ready to give yourself an injection.

Preparing a Mixed Dose of Insulin

If you take more than one type of insulin at the same time,
you can put two different types of insulin into one syringe so
that you only have to take one injection. Be sure you have
experience preparing single-dose injections before trying this
method.

1. Write down how much of each type of insulin you need.
   Write your dose of short-acting
   insulin here: _____ (A units)
   Write your dose of intermediate or
   long-acting insulin here: _____ (B units)
   Write your total dose here: _____ (A + B)
2. Clean the tops of both bottles with an alcohol swab.
3. Inject _____ (B) units of air into the longer-acting insulin bottle. *Do not* pull insulin into the syringe. Take
   the needle out of the bottle.
3. Inject _____ (A) units of air into the short-acting bottle. Turn the bottle and syringe upside down. Hold the
   bottle with one hand and use the other hand to pull the
   plunger back until you have _____ (A) units of short-
   acting insulin in the syringe. Be sure to check for air
   bubbles. (See step 8 of the previous section.)
4. Gently roll or agitate the insulin in the longer-acting
   bottle.
5. Insert the needle into the bottle of longer-acting insulin. Turn the bottle and syringe upside down. With
   the bottle in one hand, gently pull down on the
   plunger with the other until the tip of the plunger
   reaches _____ (A + B) units. Be sure not to push
   any of the short-acting insulin into the bottle. If you
   pull too much of the longer-acting insulin into the

syringe, discard the dose and start the process again
with the empty syringe.
6. Remove the needle from the bottle and you are ready
for your injection.

Giving an Insulin Injection

Giving yourself an insulin shot will probably be a little
nerve-racking at first. You probably have already given an
insulin injection under supervision or had it given to you so
you may already have a sense of what the injection feels like.

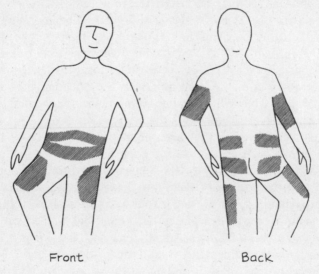

Front   Back

The Most Comfortable and Suitable Places for an Injection

*(Always give injections into fatty tissue,
never directly into an artery or vein)*

The first step is to choose an injection site. The illustration
will give you an idea of the most comfortable and suitable
places for injection; you may need a family member to give

your shot in some of the areas shown here. You should be aware that insulin is absorbed into the bloodstream faster from some areas of the body than from others. The area with the fastest rate of absorption is the abdomen, followed by the arms, then the legs. Insulin is taken up most slowly from the buttocks.

You should choose a different site (at least one inch apart) each time you give yourself an injection. This helps keep the skin, fat, and muscle healthy. Your doctor or diabetes educator will probably recommend that you rotate your injection sites by following a regular pattern, known as *site rotation*. For instance, you may be instructed to use alteRnatelimbs or to alternate injections from one side of the abdomen or buttocks to the other. This helps keep your blood sugar level more even from day to day. If you take more than one shot each day, use a different area for each shot. Start in a corner of one area and move down or across the injection sites systematically. This will help you remember where you took your last shot. After all the sites in one area have been used, you can start over in that area or move to another.

Once you have chosen an injection site, clean the skin at the site with an alcohol swab. Some people find it easier to pinch up a large area of skin, but this is not necessary with modern insulin syringes and needles. Your goal is to inject the insulin into a layer of fatty tissue just below the skin but above the muscle. Push the needle into the skin, keeping the needle between a forty-five- and a ninety-degree angle. Now release any pinched skin and push the plunger all the way down. Pull the needle straight out. Don't rub the place where you gave yourself the shot, as this could cause the insulin to be absorbed too quickly. Press your hand gently over the spot for a minute if there is any blood.

After you have given yourself an injection, properly dispose of your syringe. The safest way to do this is to place the *uncapped* syringe in a thick plastic bottle or jug, such as an empty bleach or liquid laundry detergent bottle that can be sealed shut. *(Don't* try to recap the syringe before discarding it, as you could accidentally poke yourself with the needle.) Then call your local waste disposal company and ask what their rules are regarding disposal of used needles. Some pharmacies now offer a syringe disposal service for people with diabetes in which the pharmacy gives you a medical waste disposal container in exchange for a small fee. When the container is full, you return it to the pharmacy, which arranges to have the needles incinerated.

Keeping a Medication Record

It is essential that you write down how much and what kind of insulin you take, and what time you give yourself an injection. (You'll find a sample self-care diary on page 223.) This way, you and your doctor will have the information you need to determine how well your body is responding to insulin shots. You will be instructed to regularly monitor your blood sugar levels as well (see Chapter 6). Your doctor initially may also ask you to keep a record of what you eat and the amount of exercise you get, since both your food intake and level of physical activity can affect your glucose levels and hence how much insulin you should receive.

Monitoring Your Diabetes

Since diabetes often produces no symptoms, how will you know whether your food plan, exercise, or medications are working? This is where blood glucose and other monitoring tests come in. Your physician will periodically monitor your diabetes with a variety of office tests. Between doctor visits, you can keep tabs on your blood sugar levels with a number of self-monitoring tests now available.

What to Expect from Your Doctor

Your physician has two basic ways of monitoring your blood glucose levels:

Random blood glucose test. This is the same blood glucose test used to diagnose diabetes. The test involves having blood drawn from your arm either before or after a meal to measure your blood glucose levels.

Glycosylated hemoglobin test. Because blood glucose levels vary widely over the course of a day, a single blood glucose measurement in itself is seldom a reliable indication of overall diabetes control. This is where the glycosylated hemoglobin test comes in. This test, also known as the hemoglobin A1C test, measures the amount of sugar that has attached to the hemoglobin portion of the body's red blood cells over the previous one- to two-month period. The amount that attaches is proportional to the average blood sugar level. Because red blood cells travel in the bloodstream for a total of about four months, doctors have a natural "marker" to help determine long-term blood sugar levels.

The measurement derived from the glycosylated hemoglobin test functions in much the same way as a baseball player's batting average: while a ball player might hit a home run one day and strike out the next, neither is an indication of his overall batting average, which is obtained over a long period. In the same way, blood sugar levels may be high during one blood glucose measurement and low during the next. By using the glycosylated hemoglobin test, your doctor can learn your *average* blood sugar reading, and adjust your diabetes care plan accordingly.

The test involves having blood drawn out of your arm. (There are no dietary restrictions.) The blood is then sent to a laboratory for analysis. A hemoglobin A1C test value over 9.5 percent usually indicates poorly controlled or uncontrolled diabetes. People without diabetes have values below 6.5 percent.

The American Diabetes Association recommends that all patients who receive insulin shots and those whose blood sugar levels are not under good control receive the test at least every three months; people with mild cases of diabetes can expect to be tested every six months.

Tests Available for Home Use

A number of home tests are available to help monitor your condition, including self-monitoring blood glucose (SMBG) test kits, urine glucose tests, and urine tests to detect ketones.

Self-Monitoring of Blood Glucose

As you know, your blood sugar levels are an important barometer of how well your diabetes care plan is working—so important, in fact, that monitoring your blood sugar levels regularly with self-monitoring blood-glucose (SMBG) test kits has become an integral part of diabetes management. By testing your blood sugar, you can (with the knowledge and help of your doctor) adjust your eating, exercise, and medication to maintain target blood sugar levels and keep close tabs on your condition.

Blood glucose monitoring is especially important for those who are insulin-dependent, for pregnant women with diabetes, and for those who have frequent or severe hypoglycemic reactions. But because even a well-established plan can be disrupted by illness, stress, or a change in routine, such as when you travel, all people with diabetes should be trained to test their blood sugar levels.

All SMBG tests work in roughly the same way: A small drop of blood is obtained from your fingertip, usually with a lancing device that makes it easier to prick your fingertip. The drop of blood is then applied to a chemical test strip, which changes color according to the amount of glucose in the blood. You can then "read" the results in one of two ways:

Visual testing, developed in the late 1970s, relies on test strips that change colors when they come into contact with sugar. After applying a drop of blood to the pad on the strip, you must wait the exact amount of time indicated in the instructions. (If you don't wait long enough or wait too long, the test results may be inaccurate.) You then wipe the drop of blood from the test strip according to the kit's instructions. After another waiting period, you compare the color on the chemical strip to a color chart included in the kit to obtain the range of your blood sugar level. (The chart might, for example, indicate that you have a blood sugar reading between 80 and 120 mg/dl.)

Meter testing, like visual testing, relies on chemical test strips to interpret blood glucose levels. Unlike the visual system, however, meter test kits provide you with a more precise numerical measure of blood glucose levels.

Cost, convenience, and accuracy are among the factors you should take into consideration when deciding which of the methods is better for you. Generally speaking, visual test kits are less expensive, and many people are able to assess their blood sugar levels with enough accuracy for decision-making using only visual strips. But meters are more accurate and reliable.

If you opt for meter testing, you'll have to do your homework before you buy one: more than twenty-five types of meters are currently available, varying widely in cost, ease of use, and sophistication. Some meters require that you time the test, just as you would with a visual test system; others are timed automatically. Some require that you blot the blood from the test strip; others don't. Most meters now have memory capabilities so that you or your doctor or nurse can recall information on day-to-day control. These meters can also upload to computer programs for a variety of analyses. Check with your doctor or diabetes educator before you buy one. Here are some factors to consider:

Portability. All of the meters currently on the market are extremely portable, weighing less than a pound and operating on batteries. Because meters do vary in size, however, you should shop around for the one you feel most comfortable carrying.

Ease of use. Monitors also vary widely in terms of convenience and ease of use. To decide which brand is best for you, check such factors as the number of steps required to operate the system, and whether or not you need to manually blot blood or time the procedure. If possible, try several monitors before you buy one. Your physician or diabetes educator can help you in this area, as these professionals are probably familiar with a number of different glucose monitoring systems on the market. You should make sure your doctor or nurse knows how to operate the system you select; if not, you may not use the system to its full potential.

Cost. Blood glucose meters also differ greatly in terms of cost, so it's a good idea to do some comparison shopping before making a final selection. Rebates and special-purchase offers are often available for blood glucose meters; keep an eye on advertisements and sales circulars to find the best buy.

Although many health insurance companies will pay for blood glucose monitors and equipment, some will not. Do not assume that your insurance company will reimburse you; contact your insurance carrier before making your purchase.

Also take into consideration the cost of testing supplies, such as chemical strips, control solutions, and other materials, which can become costly over time. The number of tests you will need to conduct each day will determine your overall glucose monitoring budget.

Calibration. This keeps the monitor (and hence your test results) accurate. Some monitors provide automatic calibration; others must be calibrated every so often by you.

Batteries. Some monitors are powered by regular alkaline batteries. Others run on money-saving rechargeable batteries. Still others are powered by nonreplaceable batteries that are good for a minimum of 4,000 tests.

Cleaning and maintenance. As with any type of equipment, blood glucose monitors will require some cleaning and maintenance, and some monitors need more than others.

Read and compare the manufacturer's care instructions for several models before making a decision.

Extra features. In recent years, blood glucose monitoring devices have grown increasingly sophisticated. One of the most popular "extras" now available is the data management system, which can be purchased separately and is customized for a particular memory meter. Data management systems automatically store hundreds of test results, eliminating the need for manual record-keeping. (See "The Importance of Record-Keeping," page 100.) These systems store the glucose results, time, date, and insulin type and dose. Among the many advantages of a data management system is that the information collected can be plotted on a graph, enabling you to more easily make decisions about your diabetes control based on your glucose levels over long periods.

If you decide to purchase a data management system, remember that you will need one that is compatible with your blood glucose monitor (if it is purchased separately from the monitor) as well as with your computer or your doctor's computer. If the two systems can't communicate with one another, you won't be able to retrieve the information from the data management system. Before you purchase a data management system, you should also ask your doctor what information about your treatment plan he or she needs you to record. Keep in mind, too, that data management systems are a luxury, not a necessity. Discuss the pros and cons of owning one of these systems with your physician or diabetes educator before you buy one, and shop around to ensure that you get the right system for your needs.

Urine Tests for Sugar and Ketones

Until about fifteen years ago, urine testing was the only means available for people with diabetes to check their diabetes control. However, this method of testing has a number of limitations. The chief drawback is that urine testing does not reflect current blood sugar levels; blood sugar concentrations may have been elevated anywhere from minutes to hours before the urine was collected. Consequently, a urine test could show negative results when blood glucose has actually gone back up to high levels or be positive when the glucose level is normal or low. For this reason, urine testing is not the preferred means of keeping tabs on blood glucose levels, (although it may be adequate for some persons with non-insulin-dependent diabetes who do not take insulin). Urine testing is still the only way to measure ketones, which, like glucose, build up in the blood and then spill over into the urine.

Urine glucose tests come in three basic forms: tapes, tablets, and test strips. Tapes and test strips for glucose and ketones work in much the same way as those used in blood glucose test kits. After placing the test strip or tape in a urine sample, you must wait an allotted period before "reading" the color change by comparing it with a color chart. Tablets for glucose testing are placed in a test tube with a mixture of urine and water. The tablet for ketones is read after a drop of urine is placed on it; a purple color indicates the presence of ketones.

Results of urine tests can be affected by many factors. For instance, high doses of vitamin C can skew the results, as can certain antibiotics. The test materials are sensitive to light, temperature extremes, and moisture, so be sure to store them in a cool, dry place. Check the expiration date on the package before you buy these products, and don't use the products if the initial color comparison doesn't match.

Urine tests that measure only sugar or ketones are cheaper than those that measure both. Since it is only necessary to measure urine ketones when blood sugar levels are high and with illness, it makes the most sense to use ketones-only strips or tablets. The tablets and foil-wrapped strips are more reliable; unwrapped strips lose their sensitivity rapidly after the bottle is opened.

The American Diabetes Association each year publishes a Buyer's Guide listing all currently available brands of blood glucose meters and urine tests, as well as other equipment. To obtain a copy, write to the American Diabetes Association. (See the recommended resources on page 187 for the address.)

Who Should Be Monitored, and How Often?

The frequency with which you will need to monitor your blood glucose depends on a number of factors, including the type and amount of medication you use, whether or not you are ill, and the way your medication is administered. Your physician or diabetes educator can help you determine the schedule that is best for your needs. Here are some general guidelines:

You should monitor your blood sugar levels *three to six times per day* if you

- take more than two insulin shots per day
- use an insulin pump
- are pregnant
- are ill
- are having problems with very low blood sugar

If you do not fall into one of the categories above, you can probably monitor your blood glucose levels less often. *But you will generally need to perform at least two tests per day to provide sufficient information to help you adjust your medication and food plan accordingly.* The American Diabetes Association recommends that you conduct additional tests before, during, and after exercise to help avoid hypoglycemia.

Generally speaking, you should check your blood sugar levels before breakfast, before lunch, before dinner, and at bedtime. (If you usually have a snack in the evening, measure your blood glucose *before* eating the snack.) It's also a good idea occasionally to test your blood sugar about two hours after eating. In addition, you may want to vary testing times for a few days to learn what your blood glucose patterns are during the course of an entire day.

Whenever you are sick or under stress, or undergo a major change in your routine, try to monitor your blood glucose more frequently—at least four times a day. Blood glucose levels tend to vary greatly from usual levels under these circumstances.

If you are insulin-dependent, you should also test for ketones whenever your blood sugar level is over 240 mg/dl; if you are sick with a cold, the flu, or an infection; if you are vomiting or feel sick to your stomach; if you have symptoms of high blood sugar or ketoacidosis (see Chapter 7); if you are pregnant; or if you are under extreme stress.

The Importance of Record-Keeping

Whether or not you decide to purchase a data management system, you will still need to establish a diabetes diary to keep track of your blood sugar readings. These records will ultimately help you and your physician to spot any problems in your diabetes care plan and make necessary adjustments to correct them. Your diabetes diary should contain the following information, recorded each day:

- the date
- the time your blood glucose tests were conducted
- the test results
- the time you took medication (insulin or oral medication)

- the type and dosage of the medication
- ketone test time and results
- any factors that may have altered your blood sugar level, such as increased physical activity, skipping a meal, etc. (You can make your own diary, use the one provided on page 223, or use one of the diary books available from various sources.)

Self-monitoring is an integral part of diabetes management today. But when blood sugar levels swing wildly up and down or remain high despite your best efforts at following your diabetes care plan, testing your blood sugar can become a real source of frustration—so much so, in fact, that children (and even some adults) may be tempted to falsify the results they record in their diabetes diaries. You may even be tempted to stop following your diabetes care plan, telling yourself, "What's the use? It's not working anyway!"

First, remember that a single blood sugar measurement *is not* a reliable barometer of overall diabetes control. In fact, one of the first things your doctor or diabetes educator will look for (you can, too) is a pattern of highs and lows in your blood sugar levels. If a pattern emerges, often the cause of the swings becomes more evident. For instance, in schoolchildren, often the highest blood sugar readings of the day are registered in the afternoon, just as school is letting out. This doesn't necessarily mean that the child is eating candy bars on the way home from school. It could be that the child's last class of the day is the most stressful, or that the stresses that have been building up all day reach their peak when it's time to go home. It could also reflect an inadequate insulin effect at that time of day, requiring a dose adjustment.

At any rate, blood sugar monitoring should not be viewed as a gauge of your success or failure at achieving diabetes control. Rather, you should think of monitoring as a way of determining whether or not further adjustments need to be made in your diabetes care plan.

CHAPTER 7

Emergencies

If you have insulin-dependent diabetes or if you take insulin or pills for non-insulin-dependent diabetes, you must learn how to recognize and prevent two common complications: *hypoglycemia*, or low blood sugar, and *diabetic ketoacidosis*, dangerously elevated blood sugar levels that could lead to a coma and even death. Since both of these conditions can cause you to pass out, other family members, coworkers, your travel and exercise partners, or your child's teachers and caregivers should read this chapter, too, so they'll know how to help.

Hypoglycemia

Anyone taking insulin or oral diabetes medication can experience episodes of hypoglycemia, also known as an *insulin reaction* or *insulin shock*. If you take insulin, you may experience minor episodes as often as once every two weeks. And one out of four or five insulin-dependent people will experience a severe episode every year. Hypoglycemia is also fairly common if you take oral hypoglycemic medications. Older people who take long-acting agents are particularly susceptible.

As you may recall, glucose is a major source of nutrition for your brain. When blood sugar concentrations fall below the normal range, your brain doesn't get the nutrients it needs and can't function properly. Most people with diabetes experience some unpleasant symptoms when their blood sugar level drops below 70 mg/dl. Symptoms accompanying mild hypoglycemia are usually physical. You may experience excessive hunger, break out in a sweat, feel shaky, and experience heart palpitations. If you have a moderate reaction, you may develop a headache, notice numbness or tingling in your mouth and lips, and feel confused, irritable, or drowsy. If low blood sugar is left untreated, you may even experience convulsions or pass out (coma).

Mild hypoglycemia is more of a minor annoyance than a major medical emergency. Because mild hypoglycemia makes you feel excessively hungry, you may overeat. This may lead you to gain weight or develop rebound hyperglycemia. Moderate and severe hypoglycemic episodes are more serious. Because hypoglycemia interferes with your ability to think and reason, it may be difficult for you to perform even simple mental tasks, such as balancing a checkbook. Taking a test at school may become impossible. If you experience an episode while riding a bicycle, driving a car, or operating heavy machinery, you could become a danger to yourself and others. And while hypoglycemia rarely results in death, repeated or prolonged hypoglycemic episodes may cause central nervous system damage, particularly in very young children. Repeated bouts of hypoglycemia can also erode your morale and that of your family.

Hypoglycemia is not the only cause of headaches, hunger, mood swings, or weakness, and it's often easy to overlook or ignore these early warning signs, especially if you are distracted by some other activity. A hypoglycemic episode may also be difficult to detect while you are asleep. (Signs for your family to watch for when you are asleep include noisy breathing, crying out, pallor, and sweating.) If you've had diabetes for a number of years, if you take drugs known as *beta blockers* to control high blood pressure, or if you take intensive insulin therapy, you may be at a greater risk of developing *hypoglycemic unawareness*. This condition occurs when the early warning signs, such as excessive hunger, shakiness, and sweating, become less noticeable, making serious episodes harder to detect and prevent. That's why it is essential that you regularly monitor your blood sugar levels.

Preventing Hypoglycemia

If you experience a hypoglycemic episode, you can usually pinpoint the problem by reviewing your activities in the hours just before your reaction. Understanding what triggers an episode can help you prevent further reactions.

The most common causes of hypoglycemic episodes are

- taking too much insulin or diabetes medication
- taking your medication later than usual (often as a result of sleeping late)
- skipping, delaying, or not finishing meals or snacks
- getting more exercise than usual

Another common cause of hypoglycemia is use of alcohol, marijuana, or other drugs. These substances may mask your awareness of hypoglycemia's early warning signs. Alcohol also interferes with your liver's normal ability to release glucose when blood sugar levels are low. Indeed, some of the most severe hypoglycemic reactions occur during or after parties.

Now that you know the most common causes of hypoglycemia, here are some tips for preventing a reaction:

Eat your meals on time. Don't skip meals or snacks. (If you do, don't wait for the scheduled next snack or meal if you're more than a little hungry.)

Take your diabetes medication as directed. Double-check your dosage, and take your medicine on time. What if you sleep late? Most people can safely sleep an extra thirty to forty-five minutes without a problem. One way to handle a longer delay is to get up at your usual time, test your blood sugar level, take your insulin, eat breakfast, and then go back to sleep. Whatever you do, *don't get up and take your insulin without eating, then go back to bed.* This could trigger a dangerous hypoglycemic episode.

When exercising, always carry orange juice, hard candy, or some other quick-acting carbohydrate with you. If you experience early signs of hypoglycemia during your workout, stop exercising and eat an appropriate high-carbohydrate snack. (Ask your physician or nutrition counselor what and how much you should eat in such situations.) If in the past you have experienced a hypoglycemic reaction while exercising, you can prevent a recurrence by snacking before, during, or just after exercising.

Another alternative is to adjust your insulin dosage to match your level of activity. For instance, if you normally take a short-acting insulin before breakfast but plan to exercise after breakfast, your doctor may advise you to reduce your insulin dose by 10 to 20 percent. *Don't take matters into your own hands, however. Always discuss any changes in your insulin medication with your physician beforehand.*

Monitor your blood sugar levels more frequently whenever there are changes in your insulin injections or in your eating or exercise schedules, when traveling, or when taking additional medications that may contribute to hypoglycemia. (See page 72 for a list.) If you have no symptoms but blood sugar tests detect low blood sugar levels, you should treat the condition anyway.

Treating Mild Hypoglycemic Reactions

If you have mild symptoms of hypoglycemia, test your blood. If your blood sugar level is less than 70 mg/dl or the level set by your doctor, you can usually raise your blood sugar levels quickly by eating something containing sugar. (If you can't test your blood and feel as though you are having a mild hypoglycemic episode, eat sugar-containing foods anyway.) Some likely choices:

- four to 6 ounces of a regular, carbonated *(not sugar-free)* soft drink or unsweetened fruit juices (apple or orange juice)
- five to six Life Savers or other small hard candies
- one tablespoon of honey or Karo syrup
- four teaspoons or packets of granulated sugar, or six half-inch sugar cubes
- three commercially prepared glucose tablets

Glucose gel products, which are applied between the cheek and gum, or small tubes of cake frosting work well for small children. You should avoid using chocolate and ice cream, however; the fat content of these foods could slow the body's absorption of sugar and contribute to weight problems.

If you don't feel better within fifteen minutes, eat the same amount of food again. Remember: you should eat these foods *in addition to* your regular meals and snacks. Don't change the times of your regular meals and snacks.

If you experience a hypoglycemic reaction during the night, you should consume one of the above, followed by a carbohydrate- and protein-containing snack, such as an

8-ounce glass of milk, or a 4-ounce glass of milk along with a few crackers.

If you experience mild hypoglycemia while driving, you should stop, treat it, and wait ten to fifteen minutes to make sure you have fully recovered before you resume driving.

Treating Moderate Hypoglycemic Reactions

If you have a moderate hypoglycemic reaction, you can eat any of the foods listed above, but you may require more than one treatment and it may take you longer to recover fully. (If family members or friends find you too uncooperative to eat, they may need to give you an injection of glucagon. For more on this drug, see "Treating Severe Hypoglycemia," below.)

Treating Severe Hypoglycemia

If your blood sugar level falls so low that you pass out or can't swallow, you will need a glucagon injection. This injection releases sugars stored in the liver in the same way that glucagon secreted from the pancreas does, thus rapidly raising your blood sugar level.

If you take insulin, you should *always* keep glucagon on hand. Your physician will give you a prescription for a glucagon emergency kit, which contains a bottle of glucagon and a syringe filled with a special solution. You should make sure that your family, friends, coworkers, and exercise partners know how to give glucagon since, in an emergency, you won't be able to inject it yourself. (See the instructions that follow.) Giving a glucagon injection is similar to giving an insulin injection, so have family members, friends, coworkers, exercise partners, or your child's caregivers practice by giving an insulin injection. If family, friends, coworkers, or caregivers ever find you passed out, they should give you glucagon—even if they are not sure that your blood sugar level is low.

How to Prepare and Give a Glucagon Injection

First, remove the flip-off seal from the bottle of glucagon. Now remove the cover from the syringe and inject the entire contents of the syringe into the bottle of glucagon. Remove the syringe and gently shake the bottle or roll it between the palms of your hands until the glucagon dissolves and the solution becomes clear. *Do not use the glucagon unless the solution is clear and of water-like consistency.*

Using the same syringe, withdraw the appropriate amount of the solution from the bottle. Ask your doctor or use the general guidelines here:

Age	Dosage
Under 5	0.25 to 0.50 mg
5 to 10	0.50 to 1 mg
Over 10	1 mg

You do not need to use an alcohol swab to clean the injection site unless it is visibly dirty. Insert the needle at the injection site on either the upper arm or the thigh and inject the glucagon solution. Apply light pressure at the injection site and withdraw the needle.

After giving the injection, turn the person on his or her side. This prevents choking should he or she vomit after awakening. (Some people get nauseated from glucagon.)

The person should revive within ten to fifteen minutes after getting a glucagon injection. Once the person is awake and able to swallow, he or she should be fed a fast-acting source of sugar, such as a regular soft drink or orange juice, followed by a longer-acting source of carbohydrate, such as cheese and crackers or a meat sandwich.

If the person doesn't revive within fifteen minutes, he or she should get another dose of glucagon and *emergency help should be called immediately*. Severe hypoglycemia can be life-threatening if not treated promptly.

If hypoglycemia is extremely severe or prolonged, it may take several hours for you to completely recover. If you suffered convulsions, you may develop a severe headache, feel lethargic, experience amnesia (loss of memory), or be sick to your stomach. You may also experience poor muscle control, which should be evaluated by a doctor if it persists longer than a couple of hours.

Warning Signs of Hypoglycemia

Symptoms	What to do
Mild:	
Unusual hunger	Eat or drink something
Shakiness	containing sugar:
Sweating	-regular soda or juice
Weakness	-5 or 6 small hard candies
Heart palpitations	-3 glucose tablets
	-1 tablespoon honey
	-1 tablespoon sugar or
	5 small sugar cubes
Moderate:	
Headache	Eat or drink something
Irritability	containing sugar (see
Confusion	above list)
Weakness	Place as much glucose
	gel between cheek and gum
	as possible
	Give glucagon injection if
	eating is refused

Severe:

Convulsions	Give glucagon injection
Unconsciousness	Call for emergency help
	if person can't be revived
	15 minutes after injection
	or if having a convulsion

Having an insulin reaction is a scary experience. Some people with diabetes dread it so much that they make the mistake of not taking enough insulin. This is a dangerous way to deal with hypoglycemia, because persistently elevated blood sugar levels can increase your risk of developing long-term complications (see Chapter 8) and can even lead to diabetic ketoacidosis, a much more serious medical emergency than mild hypoglycemia (see page 111). If you are having trouble with hypoglycemia, tell your doctor, who can adjust your insulin dosage if necessary. You may also want to monitor your blood sugar levels more often to help prevent a hypoglycemic episode.

Hyperglycemia

High blood sugar levels—above 240 mg/dl—are a common problem among people with diabetes. Blood sugar levels can rise slowly over a matter of days or can shoot up quickly, and usually occur after you've eaten a big meal or when you're getting sick. Your blood sugar can also rise when you're under stress or don't get your normal amount of exercise.

The symptoms of hyperglycemia are the same as those you may have experienced when you found out you had diabetes: excessive thirst, excessive hunger, frequent urination (especially at night), dry or itchy skin, fatigue, vision problems, infection, or sustaining a cut or sore that heals slowly.

High blood sugar is not life-threatening in itself, although prolonged hyperglycemia can lead to long-term complications (see Chapter 8). High blood sugar levels may progress to a life-threatening coma, a condition known as diabetic ketoacidosis in insulin-dependent people and a condition called *hypersomolar coma* in people with non-insulin-dependent diabetes (see below). For this reason, you should do everything you can to ensure that your blood sugar levels remain within a safe range. Essentially, this means following your diabetes care plan. Remember to

- eat your meals and snacks according to your meal plan and at the appropriate times
- take the prescribed amount of diabetes medication
- check your blood sugar level regularly—at least twice a day if you have non-insulin-dependent diabetes and up to four times a day if you are insulin-dependent
- record all of your test results and look for patterns of high blood sugar levels
- exercise regularly, and test your blood sugar level before and after exercising as necessary
- if you are insulin-dependent, check your urine for ketones whenever your blood sugar levels are over 240 mg/dl
- if you are ill, follow a sick-day plan (see page 154) and be extra careful to keep your fluid intake up

Diabetic Ketoacidosis and Diabetic Coma

When there isn't enough insulin in your body, it can't use the glucose circulating in your bloodstream, and blood sugar levels rise. Since your cells aren't being nourished, your body thinks it is starving. Hence, your body begins to dip into its reserve fuel supplies by converting protein into sugar and releasing fats stored in your adipose tissues into the bloodstream. But with no insulin to help these fuels enter the cells, your blood sugar levels rise even higher and *ketones*, breakdown products of fats, build up in the bloodstream. The buildup of ketones alters the delicate acid-base balance in your bloodstream, resulting in a potentially life-threatening condition known as *diabetic ketoacidosis*, or DKA. DKA usually occurs among people with insulin-dependent diabetes, but some elderly people with non-insulin-dependent diabetes may be susceptible as well. The most common cause is low insulin levels, either because you haven't yet been diagnosed with diabetes, you forgot to take an insulin injection, you didn't take enough insulin, or the insulin you took was not biologically active for some reason. One common mistake is to skip an insulin injection when you are ill, particularly when you are unable to eat. This may seem logical since you know you must eat after taking insulin when you are not sick. The stress of illness increases the liver's production of sugar and raises your blood sugar level, increasing your need for insulin. When an infection, such as pneumonia, meningitis, a stomach virus, or flu, is combined with low insulin levels, the stage is set for DKA. Trauma from an accident, a heart attack, or stroke may also trigger DKA.

DKA can develop over a few hours, particularly when you are sick with a vomiting illness. If not treated (in the hospital), it can lead to coma and even death.

If you have insulin-dependent diabetes, you should check your blood sugar and urine ketone levels whenever you experience the following symptoms: frequent urination, excessive thirst, rapid, deep breathing, dehydration (very dry mouth), a fruity smell on your breath, drowsiness, weakness, or visual disturbances. If your blood sugar is high (above 240 mg/dl) and you have ketones in your urine, call your doctor or diabetes nurse right away. He or she will tell you whether you should take more insulin and drink fluids or go to the hospital. If you are having difficulty breathing or are vomiting and cannot reach your diabetes team member, go to the emergency room of the nearest hospital immediately.

Treatment in the hospital will focus on correcting any life-threatening problems, such as dehydration, an insulin deficiency, or a potassium deficiency.

Usually, DKA can be prevented by sticking with your diabetes care plan.

• Follow your insulin routine exactly.

• Check your blood sugar levels regularly, and record the results in a diabetes diary.

• Check your urine for ketones when your blood sugar is over 240 mg/dl; when you feel sick or have a cold, the flu, or any kind of infection; when you are vomiting or feel sick to your stomach; when you have symptoms of high blood sugar or ketoacidosis; or when you are under a great deal of stress.

• Don't exercise when you have ketones in your urine and your sugar level is over 280 mg/dl.

• Contact your diabetes team as soon as you become ill, have nausea and vomiting, or have fever, or if your blood sugar levels are persistently elevated and you have ketones in your urine. When caught early, the problem can often be managed by your physician or nurse, who may recommend that you begin taking frequent injections of short-acting insulin and drink plenty of fluids. Your physician may be able to treat the condition in the emergency room of a hospital. Never continue to treat elevated glucose levels and ketones in the urine yourself if there is vomiting, rapid breathing, or a lack of response to extra insulin within a couple of hours.

Hypersomolar coma, also referred to as *hypersomolar nonketotic coma*, or more accurately, *hypoketotic coma*, occurs in people with non-insulin-dependent diabetes. It is most likely to happen to people who have limited thirst drive or access to fluids, such as people with brain injury or those who are bedridden. But almost anyone with non-insulin-dependent diabetes can develop hypersomolar coma. The problem occurs when very high blood sugar levels are combined with an inadequate amount of water in the body, resulting in decreased circulation to the brain and coma. This form of coma is treated by giving fluids intravenously.

Even though this type of coma does not affect the acid-base balance of the blood, hypersomolar coma is more dangerous than ketoacidosis and has a high mortality rate. This is why it is important to avoid dehydration when you have non-insulin-dependent diabetes.

CHAPTER 8

Long-Term Complications

The long-term complications associated with diabetes are serious and scary: heart disease; kidney disease; blindness; nerve problems that may cause pain or loss of feeling; impotence; or loss of a limb. Fortunately, most can be delayed or may even be prevented—first and foremost by maintaining good control of your diabetes. As we discussed in Chapter 1, the Diabetes Control and Complications Trial demonstrated a 60 percent reduction in risk for the development and progression of eye disease and kidney and nerve damage among study participants who maintained near-normal blood glucose levels throughout the course of the ten-year study. Although all of the study participants had insulin-dependent diabetes, the researchers are optimistic that the same tight control of diabetes will help reduce the risk of complications for people with non-insulin-dependent diabetes as well.

You should be aware, however, that the study participants were selected from a highly motivated group of people, were willing to endure frequent daily insulin injections and blood glucose tests, and were at a much greater risk of suffering hypoglycemic episodes than people receiving conventional care. Not all people with diabetes may be able to achieve such tight control of their blood sugar. Here's what you need to know about the long-term effects of diabetes on your health and what you can do to reduce the risk of serious complications.

Heart and Circulatory System

The cardiovascular system consists of the heart and some 58,000 miles of blood vessels that together are responsible for delivering oxygen and nutrients to your body's tissues and carrying away waste products. *Cardiovascular disease* is a broad term used to describe problems with the heart and blood vessels. Of particular concern to people with diabetes are two major types of cardiovascular disease: *coronary heart disease*, a progressive narrowing of the blood vessels that nourish the heart muscle, and high blood pressure, or *hypertension*—excessive force of blood on the artery walls as it is pumped through the body. Both of these can increase your risk of suffering a heart attack or stroke.

People with diabetes are also prone to develop problems with the small blood vessels *(capillaries)* that carry blood to the fingers, toes, skin, eyes, kidneys, and other parts of the body. Poorly controlled diabetes can contribute to the normal wear and tear on small blood vessels that occurs naturally with age. Diabetes also affects the connective tissue of the blood vessel wall and causes changes for the worse in fats circulating in the bloodstream, both of which can raise the risk of heart disease. High blood pressure often compounds the damage.

Let's take a closer look at coronary heart disease and hypertension, and what you can do to lower your risk of suffering a heart attack, stroke, or other complications.

Coronary heart disease: With age, everyone experiences some narrowing and hardening of the arteries, which is known as *arteriosclerosis*. In some people, this age-related change is compounded by another type of narrowing, known as *atherosclerosis*. Atherosclerosis is caused by the formation of hard plaques on the artery walls, consisting of fat deposits, calcium, fibrous material, and other substances. These plaques narrow the blood vessels, reducing the blood supply to the heart and other vital organs. If narrowing is so extensive that a blood vessel becomes totally blocked, or if a blood clot circulating in the bloodstream lodges in a narrowed artery, the blood supply to the surrounding tissues is suddenly cut off and the tissues begin to die. A heart attack occurs when this happens in the arteries that nourish the heart muscle. A stroke occurs when the blood supply leading to or in the brain becomes blocked. When the small blood vessels that nourish the hands, feet, eyes, and kidneys are affected, the reduced blood supply may cause other complications. (See the sections on "The Kidneys," "The Eyes," and "The Feet" later in this chapter.)

People with diabetes tend to develop atherosclerosis at an earlier age than people who don't have diabetes, and the blockage tends to be more severe. For this reason, diabetes is considered a major risk factor for coronary heart disease, along with high blood pressure, high cholesterol, obesity, lack of exercise, and cigarette smoking.

One reason that people with diabetes may be more susceptible to atherosclerosis is that they often have high levels of the fatty substance known as *cholesterol* circulating in their bloodstream. Moreover, people with diabetes tend to have higher levels of low-density lipoproteins (LDL cholesterol), associated with a higher risk of heart disease, and lower levels of high-density lipoproteins (HDL cholesterol), believed to protect against heart disease, than people without diabetes.

Much of the cholesterol in your body is manufactured by the liver. However, fat and cholesterol in the foods you eat— namely meats, milk, cheese, butter, and other dairy products—can contribute to the problem. Being overweight can, too. Obesity is associated with higher levels of total and LDL cholesterol and lower levels of HDL cholesterol.

Because insulin is needed for the body's tissues to efficiently absorb triglycerides (the major type of fat in our diets), people with diabetes tend to have high blood levels of triglycerides. High triglycerides are also associated with an increased risk of heart disease.

You won't know that you have high cholesterol *(hypercholesterolemia)* or high triglycerides *(hypertriglyceridemia);* these conditions do not cause any symptoms. For this reason, your physician will periodically have your blood cholesterol and other lipids tested. People with total cholesterol levels greater than 240 mg/dl are at increased risk for coronary heart disease, particularly if the HDL is low (below 35 mg/dl).

Most people with non-insulin-dependent diabetes can lower their blood cholesterol levels through diet alone. And it just so happens that the best way to control your diabetes— eating, a low-fat, high-carbohydrate, high-fiber diet—is also the best way to lower your total and LDL blood cholesterol. So if you are following your meal plan, you will likely experience a gradual lowering of total and LDL cholesterol.

If diet therapy fails to lower your blood cholesterol or triglyceride levels, your doctor may prescribe cholesterol-lowering drugs. These include *cholestyramine* (Questran); *colestipol* (Colestid); *lovastatin* (Mevacor); *simvastatin* (Zocor); *gemfibrozil* (Lopid), a prescription form of the B-vitamin niacin; or possibly *psyllium seed,* a type of dietary fiber found in over-the-counter bulk fiber laxatives, such as Metamucil.

To further lower your risk of suffering a heart attack, you should have your blood pressure checked regularly and, if you have hypertension, follow your treatment program for lowering your blood pressure (see below). Regular exercise can reduce your risk of heart disease, too. Exercise raises levels of protective HDL cholesterol, lowers your blood pressure, and may increase levels of a powerful anticoagulant in the bloodstream that can protect against the development of blood clots. If you smoke, you should quit, since cigarette smoking significantly increases your risk of suffering a heart attack.

Hypertension: For reasons not entirely understood, people with diabetes are at a greater risk of developing high blood pressure. The danger is that high blood pressure puts added strain on blood vessels throughout your body and may help trigger the development of eye disease (retinopathy), kidney disease, and atherosclerosis. If you already have one of these conditions, having hypertension can speed its progression. The increased pressure on the blood vessel walls contributes to the damage of the lining from atherosclerosis and blood clots.

Your doctor will take a blood pressure reading at least once a year, if not more often. A blood pressure reading actually consists of two numbers: the top number, or *systolic* pressure, represents the force of blood on the arteries as the heart contracts. The bottom number, *diastolic pressure*, is the blood pressure when the heart is at rest.

If you have hypertension, you will probably be advised to reduce your sodium (salt) intake, since a diet high in sodium can raise blood pressure among certain sodium-sensitive people. (For tips on reducing the sodium in your diet, see page 39.) If you are overweight, losing weight often lowers blood pressure to safer levels. Exercise is one of the best ways to help shed pounds, and exercise itself reduces blood pressure. (Check with your doctor before beginning an exercise program, however, since people with very high blood pressure may require a limited exercise program.) Drink alcohol only in moderation, since excessive consumption of alcohol—three drinks or more a day—can *raise* your blood pressure.

If diet and exercise fail to sufficiently lower your blood pressure, your doctor may prescribe one or more types of antihypertensive drugs. You should be aware that because you have diabetes, you may be more susceptible to the side effects of certain drugs used to treat hypertension, such as hypoglycemia. If you must take drugs to lower your blood pressure, your doctor will probably prescribe such anti-

hypertensive medications as ACE inhibitors or calcium chan-
nel blockers, which are associated with fewer side effects.

If you have high cholesterol (or other signs of coronary
heart disease) or high blood pressure, it's also important to
know the early warning signs of a heart attack or stroke. The
earlier you get treatment, the greater are the chances that you
will survive. According to the American Heart Association,
you should immediately call for emergency help if you experience any of the following warning signs of a heart attack:

- an uncomfortable pressure, fullness, squeezing, or pain in
  the center of the chest that does not go away in a few
  minutes
- severe chest pain
- pain that spreads to the shoulders, neck, or arms
- lightheadedness or heart palpitations
- fainting
- sweating associated with chest discomfort
- nausea associated with chest discomfort
- difficulty breathing

Call for emergency help if you experience any of these
warning signs of a stroke:

- sudden weakness or numbness of the face, arm, and leg
  on one side of the body
- loss of speech, or trouble talking or understanding speech
- dimness or loss of vision, particularly in only one eye
- unexplained dizziness, unsteadiness, or sudden falls

The Nervous System

Some of the most common and perplexing complications associated with diabetes are those affecting the central nervous

system—the sophisticated network of hardwiring (nerves) and software (hormones and other chemical messengers) that allows the brain and the body to communicate with one another. Depending on which part of the central nervous system is affected, symptoms can range from chronic pain to diarrhea to sexual problems.

No one knows exactly how the damage occurs. High sugar concentrations in the bloodstream are believed to somehow interfere with *nerve conduction* (the way in which nerves communicate with one another). Nerve damage may also be caused or worsened by poor blood circulation, which may result in inadequate delivery of nutrients and oxygen to the nerves.

Many illnesses, certain medications, chronic alcohol intake, poor nutrition, exposure to chemical toxins, and physical injury can all cause symptoms identical to those of the various types of nerve damage associated with diabetes. For this reason, your physician will have you undergo a thorough physical examination before making a diagnosis. Be sure to provide your doctor with a list of all the medications you are taking, and be candid about your alcohol consumption and diet.

Some types of nerve damage affect mainly the hands and feet, causing either intense pain (on one or both sides of the body) or a gradual loss of sensation. Early warning signs of this type of nerve damage include pain, burning, tingling, or loss of feeling in the feet or hands.

Fortunately, many of the complications that cause pain subside by themselves within several months to a year. In the meantime, your doctor may prescribe medications to help relieve symptoms, such as the antiseizure drug phenytoin (Dilantin), the analgesics carbamazepine (Tegretol) or propoxyphene (Darvon, Wygesic), the antidepressant amitriptyline (Elavil, Endep, Etrafon, Limbitrol, Pherphenazine, Triavil), or plain aspirin. Researchers are also experimenting with aldose reductase inhibitors, which block the formation of sugar alcohols thought to be involved in the nerve problems of diabetes.

You may have heard that B vitamins alleviate symptoms of nerve damage. Although B vitamins have been used extensively to treat such nerve damage, they have not been proved effective. In fact, high doses of vitamin B_6 may actually aggravate symptoms.

If you lose feeling in your feet—what is known as *insensitive feet*—the damage is usually permanent and could lead to more serious problems, even amputation due to gangrene. Gangrene occurs when insensitive feet become injured or damaged without your knowing about it and an infection develops that is not quickly treated. Since you may not be aware that you are losing sensation in your feet, your doctor will perform several tests at least once a year, includ ing tests of how well you can sense temperature, a pinprick, vibration, and the position of your toes as your doctor flexes and extends them. You should also learn how to care for your feet to prevent serious problems (see "The Feet" on page 131).

Nerve damage to the autonomic nervous system (the part you don't control, which governs hormones, your heart rate, breathing, etc.) can affect the smooth functioning of a number of different organ systems, causing a wide range of annoying symptoms. One potentially dangerous consequence of this kind of nerve damage is a decreased awareness of the symptoms of hypoglycemia, what is known as *hypoglycemia unawareness*. This means you no longer are aware of low blood sugar levels because the effects of adrenaline, which causes cold sweats, feelings of fear, and trembling associated with hypoglycemic episodes, are missing. If you develop hypoglycemia unawareness, you should monitor your blood glucose regularly, since this is the only way you will know whether your blood sugar concentrations are falling to dangerously low levels. You should also carry hard candy, glucose tablets, or another form of sugar with you at all times, and wear a necklace or bracelet stating that you have diabetes. Keep a supply of glucagon on hand and make sure your family and friends know how and when to use it. (For more on how to treat hypoglycemia, see Chapter 7, "Emergencies.")

Other types of autonomic nerve damage include the following:

Gastrointestinal system: Nausea, vomiting, abdominal discomfort, bloating, and loss of appetite may be caused by a condition known as *gastroparesis.* One of the best remedies is attaining good control of your diabetes. You may also be advised to eat small, liquid, low-fiber, low-fat meals. Your doctor may prescribe the antiheartburn, antinausea medication metoclopramide, which often brings relief.

Some people may develop *diabetic diarrhea,* characterized by abdominal cramping and frequent passage of loose stools, particularly after meals and at night. During remissions, you may experience constipation. Eating plenty of high-fiber foods and making regular efforts to move your bowels may be helpful. Your doctor may also recommend that you take an antidiarrheal medication, such as Imodium, Donnagel, or Lomotil. Sometimes a broad-spectrum antibiotic, such as tetracycline, works. Metoclopramide may also be effective.

Urinary tract: When the nerves that help control the bladder become damaged, you may have to strain to start urinating, find it difficult to completely empty your bladder, or there may be dribbling while urinating instead of a steady stream of urine. These bladder changes increase your risk of developing bladder and kidney infections which, if left untreated, could cause permanent kidney damage. A classic symptom is feeling as if you have to urinate but not being able to do so.

Treatment involves using techniques to improve bladder emptying (ask your physician). If these measures don't help, you may have to undergo surgery to correct the problem.

Heart and circulatory system: The most common problem is a fixed heart rate that doesn't vary with the demands of the rest of the body (such as when you exercise). *Orthostatic hypotension,* a drop in blood pressure when you stand or sit up that may cause dizziness and, in severe cases, may cause you to pass out, is also common.

If you develop orthostatic hypotension, your doctor may advise you to get up slowly when you sit or stand to give the blood in your legs time to circulate back toward your upper body and head. He or she may also recommend that you wear compression stockings or an abdominal binder to help keep blood from pooling in your lower body.

Reproductive system: Nerve damage involving the reproductive system may cause problems in sexual function. Damage to the nerves and blood vessels that control sensation and circulation to a man's penis may make it difficult or impossible to achieve or sustain an erection, resulting in *impotence.* The man's sex drive and ability to ejaculate are not normally affected. Men who suffer from impotence should first undergo a medical evaluation to determine whether the problem is psychological or physiological. If the cause of impotence is in fact diabetes, penile implants can help sustain an erection. These are plastic balloons that are pumped up to help the man achieve an erection. The success rate for the implants is about 90 percent. A promising new alternative treatment involves injections of substances that dilate the blood vessels in the penis. The simplest approach is a ring and suction system that is applied over the penis and fills it by creating a vacuum, then keeps the penis full by blocking the return flow of blood.

Women with diabetes may experience decreased vaginal lubrication and painful intercourse *(dyspareunia)* as a result of nerve damage. Using a vaginal lubricant often helps.

Since impotence and dyspareunia are often accompanied by performance anxiety, both partners should consider seeing a sex therapist or marriage counselor as well.

The Kidneys

Your kidneys serve as a filtering system whose job is to remove waste products from the blood. The kidneys consist of millions of closely packed small blood vessels that carry blood through the organs, where it is filtered through goblet-shaped collecting cups known as *nephrons*. Waste materials are then excreted as urine through two tubes *(ureters)* leading to the bladder. The filtered blood is circulated back into the bloodstream. The kidneys also regulate the body's water content and help control blood pressure.

Diabetic kidney disease *(nephropathy)* is one of the main causes of premature death in people with diabetes. (The other main cause is premature cardiovascular disease.) The condition is characterized by thickening of the walls of the tiny blood vessels that filter blood through the kidneys, as well as an accumulation of connective tissue in the spaces between the vessels and the nephrons. These changes are believed to result from exposure of the tissues to excess glucose. High blood pressure and kidney infections (usually resulting from an untreated bladder infection) may also damage the tiny blood vessels in the kidneys. Use of certain drugs (notably chronic use of pain relievers such as aspirin) and diagnostic X-ray tests involving contrast dyes can add to the injury. Diets high in protein can also tax the kidneys by increasing pressure on the filtering membranes.

Once the damage is done, the kidneys' ability to filter waste products from the blood is decreased. Waste products then build up in the bloodstream, and substances the body needs, such as protein, may be excreted in the urine. If left untreated, kidney disease can progress to life-threatening kidney failure and even death.

Kidney damage doesn't produce symptoms in its early stages, which is why your doctor will recommend that you undergo a urinalysis (to detect protein or albumin in the urine) and blood tests to determine kidney function when you are first diagnosed with non-insulin-dependent diabetes. (Kidney disease may already be present at the time of diagnosis among people with non-insulin-dependent diabetes. It generally develops after 10 to 15 years, and after adolescence among people with insulin-dependent diabetes.) Kidney tests should be done every year. If you are found to have protein or albumin in your urine, your doctor may recommend that you submit another urine sample so that it can be cultured in a laboratory to determine whether you have an infection. If any of these test results is abnormal, your doctor may refer you to a specialist for further evaluation and treatment.

Many kidney problems can be prevented by taking certain precautions. The most important is keeping your diabetes under control. Poor diabetes control can speed the progression of kidney disease.

You should also have your blood pressure checked regularly. High blood pressure puts added strain on the kidneys that could speed the progression of kidney disease. If you have hypertension, stick with your treatment program: follow a no-salt-added diet, keep your weight under control and, if a blood pressure medication has been prescribed for you, take it every day.

People with diabetes are more susceptible to urinary tract infections, partly because bacteria that make their way into the urinary tract thrive on high blood sugar levels, and partly because some people with diabetes experience nerve damage that makes it difficult for them to empty the bladder completely. If urinary tract infections are left untreated, they can ascend to the kidneys, causing even more damage. For this reason, you should know the symptoms of urinary tract infections and seek treatment immediately. Call your doctor whenever you experience any of the following symptoms:

- more frequent urination, particularly at night
- a burning sensation with urination
- cloudy or bloody urine

- urgency (a need to urinate right away)
- back pain, chills, and fever (these symptoms may indicate that you have a kidney infection)

If you have a urinary tract infection, your doctor will prescribe antibiotics. *(Never* try to treat a urinary tract infection yourself with such home remedies as cranberry juice.) Your doctor may have you undergo a repeat urine culture after you have been treated to ensure that the infection has been eradicated.

If you have already sustained some degree of kidney damage, your doctor will recommend that you take steps to ensure that the damage doesn't get worse. You will be advised to have your blood pressure monitored at least four times a year if you do not have hypertension. If you already have high blood pressure, you may want to test your blood pressure regularly at home between doctor visits to make sure it stays below 140/90. If you have hypertension, you must follow your treatment plan to keep it under control. You may be advised to limit the salt and protein in your diet so that the kidneys aren't overburdened. You should also ask your doctor about which medications and X-ray dyes you should avoid. Kidney dialysis and kidney transplantation are options for those suffering from severe kidney damage or kidney failure.

The Eyes

Diabetes is the leading cause of new cases of blindness in the United States. As with other serious long-term complications, controlling your diabetes is one of the most important ways in which you can help prevent serious vision problems.

You may have already experienced one of the ways in which your vision can be affected by diabetes. High blood sugar levels affect the fluid content of the lens, resulting in blurred vision or rapid changes in vision. This type of vision change is *not* permanent. In fact, once your blood sugar levels are brought under control, your vision will return to normal.

Far more serious and potentially vision-threatening is a disorder known as *diabetic retinopathy*. Almost everyone who has diabetes for fifteen years or more will have changes in the tiny capillaries that nourish the retina of the eye. For reasons that aren't clear yet, long-standing diabetes causes parts of the capillary walls to weaken and balloon outward forming tiny pockets known as *aneurysms*. Some capillaries may become blocked altogether, cutting off the blood supply to parts of the retina.

Not all of these changes are serious. You may not even notice any symptoms or change in your vision. Sometimes, however, these changes may progress to a more dangerous stage, known as *proliferative diabetic retinopathy*. When this happens, new blood vessels and fibrous tissue form in front of the retina. New blood vessels are prone to bleed, as are those weakened by the development of aneurysms. If minor bleeding occurs, you may experience "floaters" or "cobwebs" in your field of vision. If you suffer a major retinal hemorrhage, you will experience a sudden and painless loss of vision. Sometimes the fibrous tissue causes the retina to detach from the back of the eye, which can also result in sudden blindness.

Diabetic retinopathy may result in another condition known as *diabetic macular edema*, which is caused by either a thickening of the retina or the formation of a hard fatty spot near the *macula*, the area on the retina where vision is most sharp. Macular edema can cause partial vision loss or total blindness if not treated.

People with diabetes are also at a greater risk of developing other vision-threatening eye diseases, including cataracts and glaucoma. *Cataracts* are changes in the lens of the eye that turn it opaque and cause clouded vision. *Glaucoma* is increased pressure within the eye caused by an obstruction in the flow of *aqueous humor*, the clear, watery fluid that fills the eyeball, from the front chamber of the eye. The increased pressure associated with glaucoma may damage the optic nerve and cause vision disturbances (most notably tunnel vision, a narrowed field of vision) and, if left untreated, blindness.

All of these conditions can be treated, and the earlier they are caught, the less likely they will be to cause vision problems or blindness. The problem is that diabetic retinopathy—the most common eye disease among people with diabetes—rarely causes symptoms in its earliest stages. For this reason, you should undergo regular eye examinations by your physician. At least once a year, you should have your eyes examined by an ophthalmologist, who will use special drops to dilate your pupils, enabling the doctor to get a better look at the retina. If you have had insulin-dependent diabetes for five years and are older than thirteen years or have non-insulin-dependent diabetes of any duration, *you should have your eyes examined every year even if you are not having any eye or vision problems.*

Here are some other ways you can avoid serious vision problems:

• Keep your diabetes under control. Follow your meal plan, take your medication, and monitor your blood sugar levels as directed by your doctor. Population studies suggest that people whose diabetes is poorly controlled are more likely to develop diabetic retinopathy and diabetic macular edema.

• Have your blood pressure checked regularly. If you have high blood pressure, follow your treatment plan for lowering it. People with hypertension are at an increased risk of developing diabetic retinopathy and of having the disease progress to vision-threatening stages faster than people with normal blood pressure.

• If you are pregnant or are planning to get pregnant, you should have your eyes examined, preferably *before* you conceive, and certainly in the early weeks of your pregnancy. Retinopathy may progress very rapidly during pregnancy, and you should be monitored closely throughout your pregnancy.

• If you have diabetic retinopathy, avoid exercises that can aggravate the condition, such as weight lifting, isometric exercises, and activities that require your head to be lower than your midsection more than briefly, such as headstands and certain other yoga positions.

• Don't smoke. Cigarette smoking constricts the small blood vessels in the retina and can contribute to the damage.

• Report any vision problems promptly. If you experience blurred vision, double vision, tunnel vision, dark spots, or pressure or pain in your eyes, notify your doctor.

A treatment known as *laser photocoagulation* is used to treat severe diabetic retinopathy. Doctors are not sure how the treatment works, but it has a clear, direct effect: the new (proliferative) vessels are destroyed by multiple laser burns to the retina. The treatment also has an indirect effect: it prevents new vessels from forming and reduces macular edema. When initiated in the early stages of the disease, the laser treatment can reduce the risk of severe vision loss by more than 60 percent. Laser photocoagulation can also reduce the risk of moderate vision loss from macular edema by 60 percent.

If massive bleeding has occurred or if the retina has become detached, a procedure called *closed vitrectomy* can restore useful vision about 50 to 65 percent of the time. During the procedure, the vitreous fluid of the eyeball is removed and replaced with a salt solution.

Some types of cataracts—usually those that develop in young people with insulin-dependent diabetes—may lessen or disappear altogether once the diabetes is brought under control. More than likely, however, if you have cataracts, you will need to have them surgically removed. Surgery is 90 to 95 percent successful in restoring useful vision. Be sure to discuss the potential risks of surgery with your doctor before having an operation.

Treatment for glaucoma includes the use of eye drops to help relieve pressure. If eye drops are ineffective, laser surgery may be necessary.

The Feet

Poor circulation, nerve damage, and infection can cause serious foot problems for people with diabetes, problems that could even lead to amputations. Indeed, more than half of the nontraumatic amputations in the United States occur among people with diabetes. Experts estimate that two-thirds of these amputations could have been prevented with proper care.

You may be at greater risk of developing foot problems if you

- are over age forty
- smoke cigarettes
- have had diabetes for more than ten years
- have poor circulation or loss of sensation in your feet
- have physical deformities, such as bunions, hammertoes, or clawfeet (see illustration)
- have had foot ulcers or amputations in the past

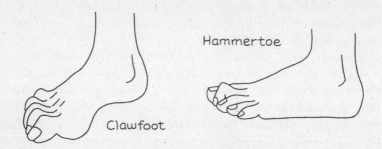

Common Foot Deformities

One of the earliest signs of trouble is *insensitive feet*, loss of feeling in the feet. When caught early, the condition is often reversible. If left untreated, however, nerve damage can shorten the tendons in the foot and lead to deformities. This, in turn, may cause you to walk differently, creating abnormal pressure points on your feet that can develop into blisters, sores, or ulcers. Another consequence of (autonomic) nerve damage in the feet is decreased sweating and skin dryness, resulting in cracked and thickened skin that could develop into an ulcer. Since the sore doesn't cause any pain, you may not even notice it. Moreover, without pain to tell you there's a problem, you may continue to walk on the sore, neglecting to give it the rest it needs to heal.

If you also have poor blood circulation in your feet, the inflamed skin and injured cells around the ulcer won't get the extra blood and nutrients they need to heal. If the wound is open, dirt and germs may get in, and the sore will easily become infected, causing more inflammation. But because you don't have adequate blood flow to the inflamed tissue, the infection spreads. If the infection spreads to the deep tissues of the body or the bone and gangrene develops, amputation may be the only recourse.

One of the best ways you can prevent this from happening is to maintain good control over your diabetes. When blood sugar levels remain in the normal range, you will be less likely to sustain the nerve and blood vessel damage that leads to foot problems.

If you already have insensitive feet, proper care of your feet can help prevent minor problems from developing into something more serious. This includes early detection and prompt treatment of any foot lesions. You may also need the help of certain specialists, including a podiatrist (foot specialist), an orthopedist (musculoskeletal specialist), a vascular surgeon, and experts in shoe fitting.

What Your Doctor Can Do

Your doctor can diagnose nerve damage to the feet by tapping your ankle with a rubber mallet to test your reflexes. He or she may also touch your foot with a cool piece of metal (such as a tuning fork) or a test tube containing cool or warm water and ask you to describe its temperature. Another test for insensitive feet involves having the doctor place a vibrating tuning fork on your foot and ask you to say when the vibration ceases. Your doctor may have you close your eyes while he or she touches the head or point of a pin to your foot, asking you to tell whether you feel a sharp or dull sensation, or no sensation at all. Finally, you may be asked to close your eyes and describe the position of your toes as your doctor alternately flexes and extends them.

Your doctor will also check your pulses in your ankles, behind your knees, and in your groin to determine whether you have adequate blood circulation.

Be sure to remove your shoes and socks during your regular diabetes checkups as a reminder to have the doctor check your feet. You should also tell your doctor about any foot or leg pain you may be experiencing while sitting, standing, or walking. This could be a sign of circulatory problems.

What You Can Do

If you have insensitive feet, poor circulation in your feet, or foot deformities, you'll need to take special care of your feet. Here are some ways in which you can help prevent an amputation:

Clean your feet. Wash your feet every day with mild soap and warm water. (Check the water temperature with your wrist, your elbow, or a thermometer—90 to 95 degrees Fahrenheit is safe.) Dry your feet with a soft towel, taking care to dry between your toes. Unless your doctor advises you otherwise, don't soak your feet; this can dry your skin, which can lead to infections. *Never* soak your feet in Epsom salts.

Soften dry skin by applying a thin coat of oil, lotion, or cream (lanolin-containing creams work well) on the tops and bottoms of your feet—not between the toes. Softening between the toes can encourage infection.

Inspect your feet. Every day after washing, inspect the tops and bottoms of your feet for cracks, blisters, bumps, infections, and injuries. Use an unbreakable mirror to check the bottoms of your feet. Don't forget to look between your toes, too. If you can't check your own feet, have someone else do it for you.

Report any sores, infections, swelling, or foot deformities to your doctor immediately. Infection can spread quickly, so prompt treatment is essential.

Give yourself a pedicure. Cut your toenails straight across and smooth the corners with an emery board. Don't trim the corners of your toenails or cut ingrown toenails. If you notice redness around the nail bed, see your doctor or podiatrist immediately.

Never use chemicals, iodine, corn plasters, razor blades, or liquid corn or callus removers to remove corns or calluses from your feet. If you have corns or calluses, have your doctor show you how to gently remove the dead skin with a pumice stone. You may want to see a foot care specialist for help with ingrown toenails, thick or yellowed nails, corns, or calluses. Ask your doctor for a referral.

Select the right shoes. Buy and wear shoes that are shaped like your feet. Shoes made of soft leather or canvas are best. From the moment you try them on in the store, make sure shoes fit comfortably and that there's plenty of room for your toes. *Don't expect new shoes to stretch out.* Avoid tight-fitting shoes or shoes with pointed toes. These can restrict blood flow to the feet. Don't wear plastic shoes, which are stiff and nonbreathing, or sandals with thongs between the toes, either. Slowly break in new shoes by wearing them only one or two hours a day.

If you have foot deformities, you will almost certainly need specially molded shoes; deformed feet will not fit into ordinary shoes, and if you have lost sensitivity in your feet, you may not even realize that regular shoes don't fit properly. Ask your doctor for a referral to a specialist in shoe fitting.

Always wear shoes with clean, thick cotton or wool socks. Don't wear mended socks. The seams could rub against your feet and cause irritation or blisters. Avoid garters that circle the leg and stockings with elastic tops; these may restrict blood flow to your feet. (For the same reason, avoid sitting with your legs crossed.)

Before putting on your shoes, look and feel inside them for loose objects, nail points, torn linings, and rough areas.

Care for your feet every day. Avoid exposing your feet to temperature extremes. Always test the water temperature with your wrist, elbow, or a bath thermometer before bathing. Always wear shoes and socks when you walk on hot surfaces, such as sand at the beach. In summer, apply sunscreen to the tops of your feet. In winter, wear wool socks and footwear such as fleece-lined boots. If your feet are cold at night, wear socks. Don't use hot-water bottles, heating pads, or other electrical devices to keep your feet warm; they could burn your feet.

Don't walk barefoot, even in the house. Wearing shoes and socks, even when indoors, protects you from stubbing your toe, stepping on a sharp object or hot surface, and other injuries.

Avoid circulatory and nerve problems. If you smoke cigarettes, quit. Even one cigarette can cause blood vessels to constrict for an hour or longer, decreasing blood circulation. If you have high blood pressure or high cholesterol, work with your doctor to lower it. Avoid excessive alcohol consumption as well. Alcohol can cause hypoglycemia without warning symptoms, and further damage nerve function.

Treat foot injuries. Attend to minor wounds promptly. Clean the area with soap and water and dry it thoroughly. Apply a nonirritating antiseptic solution and cover it with clean gauze or a bandage. Change the dressing every day. Stay off your feet as much as you can.

If a wound seems to heal slowly, or if you notice inflammation, swelling, or a break in the skin, see your doctor immediately. You should also be familiar with the warning signs of foot problems.

Warning Signs of Foot Problems

Notify your doctor if you notice any of the following:

- cold feet
- pain in the calf or foot when you are sitting, standing, or walking
- pain when you are resting your feet, particularly at night
- Burning, tingling, or crawling sensations in your feet, pain and hypersensitivity
- weakness
- diminished sweating, dry skin
- a gradual change in the shape of your foot

- a sudden, painless change in your foot shape, usually accompanied by swelling
- exquisitely painful injuries; painless wounds
- slow-healing wounds or wounds that won't heal
- changes in the color of the skin (redness or a bluish discoloration of the skin)
- frequent infections, such as athlete's foot, or inflammation (redness) of the tissue surrounding the toenails

Teeth and Gums

High blood sugar levels make people with diabetes more susceptible to *periodontal disease*, the medical term for gum disease. *Gingivitis*, inflammation of the soft tissues surrounding the teeth, is an early and reversible form of gum disease. If left untreated, gingivitis may progress to periodontitis, an infection of the supporting ligaments and bony socket of the tooth, which can eventually lead to tooth loss. Having gum disease can raise your blood sugar levels even higher.

Gum disease is caused by the bacteria in *plaque*, a sticky, nearly invisible film that constantly forms on teeth and gums. If plaque is not removed from your teeth regularly, the bacteria begin producing toxins that inflame the gums and damage the supporting ligaments and bony sockets of the teeth.

Gum disease rarely causes pain and can easily go undetected, which is why regular visits to the dentist are a must. Some telltale signs of gingivitis are bleeding gums when you brush your teeth, a bad taste in your mouth, or swollen, red gums. More advanced gum disease may cause such symptoms as oral pain, loose teeth, or difficulty in chewing. Your dentist can look for signs of periodontal disease during regular checkups. Dental X rays can help diagnose bone damage, and a tool called a periodontal probe can be used to measure the depth of pockets that form between the teeth and gums, which can help determine the extent of the disease.

Preventing gum disease is much easier than having the surgery often required to treat it. Here are a few pointers:

- Brush your teeth at least twice a day (once before bedtime). Use a soft toothbrush and toothpaste with fluoride. (Tartar-control toothpastes are of limited use, since they only remove tartar [hardened plaque] above the gumline; this plays little role in the development of gum disease.) To help keep bacteria from growing on your toothbrush, rinse it after each brushing and store it with the bristles at the top. Replace your toothbrush every three months (sooner if the bristles mat or splay).

- Floss or clean between your teeth at least once a day. This is needed to remove plaque that builds up between your teeth (where the brush can't reach) and at the gumline. If you find flossing difficult, talk to your dentist or dental hygienist about other methods of cleaning between your teeth, such as bridge cleaners, water sprayers, or special soft wood toothpicks.

- See your dentist at least every six months (more often if you have periodontal disease). While brushing and flossing can remove plaque above the gumline, a professional cleaning is needed to remove plaque and tartar that accumulate just under the gumline. Your dentist can help show you the proper way to brush and floss your teeth, and can prescribe antiplaque rinses if necessary.

You should make a dental appointment right away if you have any of the signs of gum disease (bad breath, a bad taste in your mouth, swollen, red gums, bleeding or sore gums, sore or loose teeth, or difficulty chewing). Gum disease can progress rapidly, and with advanced disease, extensive tooth loss can ^{occur} over a matter of months. And while it is possible to get dentures if you lose teeth to peri-odontitis, dentures often fit poorly over gums damaged by periodontitis. The resulting discomfort may limit your di-etary choices and in this way interfere with your diabetes management. Remember, too, that the infection itself can raise your blood sugar levels, as can the dental procedures needed to treat advanced periodontitis, which can also wreak havoc with your diabetes control.

Plan your dental appointments so that they don't inter-fere with your medication and meal schedule. Just after breakfast may be a good time. And don't skip meals or di-abetes medication before your appointment.

Be sure to remind your dentist or dental hygienist that you have diabetes. Your dentist should have the name and telephone number of your diabetes health care provider; he or she may need to consult with the physician about the management of your dental problem in relation to the dia-betes or need to call if a problem occurs while you are at the dentist's office.

• Keep your diabetes under control. High blood sugar levels speed the progression of gum disease.

Whether you are a patient with diabetes or a parent or caregiver of someone with diabetes, the condition places an enormous responsibility on you. As a result, if complications develop later in life, it's natural to blame yourself. You should know that while the tools we have available to treat diabetes are much, much better than they were even ten years ago, and are improving every day, they are not ade-quate to completely prevent many of the long-term complica-tions of the disease. These complications are tough enough to deal with without feeling that you should have been able to prevent them. On the other hand, we do know that people who have very poor diabetes control develop complications earlier than those with better control. The best you can do, then, is to work to achieve the best control possible for you.

CHAPTER 9

Pregnancy

Before insulin was developed, women with diabetes were usually too ill to conceive, let alone carry a baby to term. For the rare woman who did manage to conceive a child, the pregnancy typically ended in tragedy: the fetus usually died, and often, so did the mother. Today the fetal survival rate for women with diabetes (97 percent) is almost the same as that for mothers who don't have diabetes (98 to 99 percent). It is almost unheard of for women with diabetes to die in childbirth or to die later on of complications arising from the birth of the baby. Nevertheless, diabetes *does* increase certain risks for mother and baby. With a good understanding of the possible risks, you'll be better able to help prevent them.

Possible Risks to the Mother

In order to provide the fetus with a continuous supply of fuel during pregnancy, the body's processing of carbohydrates is altered. Many of the normal hormonal changes of pregnancy cause insulin resistance. To keep blood sugar levels normal, the body has to produce more insulin as the pregnancy progresses. Therefore, insulin levels are much higher during pregnancy in women who don't have diabetes.

If you have diabetes (either insulin-dependent or non-insulin-dependent), these normal pregnancy-related changes increase your risk of hypoglycemia, hyperglycemia, and diabetic ketoacidosis. In the early months, you may be at a greater risk of experiencing hypoglycemia, particularly if morning sickness keeps you from eating as you should. Hypoglycemic episodes may be more of a problem at night, when you are not eating for a longer period.

In the last third of pregnancy, when insulin resistance is highest, your insulin needs may rise as much as 50 percent over a matter of weeks. The increased demands of pregnancy on your body at this time also raise your risk of experiencing hyperglycemia and diabetic ketoacidosis. These problems can often be avoided by diligently monitoring your blood sugar levels throughout your pregnancy. (More on self-monitoring later.)

What about eye disease? If you don't already have diabetic retinopathy, you probably will not develop it during pregnancy. A few women with background retinopathy at the start of pregnancy may experience some worsening of the condition, but it rarely progresses to the vision-threatening proliferative stage (in which new blood vessels form). Even if you have proliferative retinopathy, the condition usually doesn't worsen during pregnancy *as long as you undergo laser photocoagulation and the retinopathy is stable before you get pregnant. Women at greatest risk of developing serious vision problems during pregnancy are those with proliferative diabetic retinopathy that has not been treated with laser photocoagulation.*

Kidney problems may temporarily worsen during pregnancy, too, since the mother's increased blood volume during pregnancy puts an added strain on the kidneys. Typically, any worsening of kidney disease clears up after delivery. But if you have advanced kidney disease, particularly if you also have hypertension, you are at a much greater risk of developing *preeclampsia.* This is a condition of high blood pressure together with protein in the urine and water retention *(edema)* that develops during the last part of pregnancy. If left untreated, this condition can damage the mother's nervous system, blood vessels, or kidneys, and can cause a slowing of growth or lack of oxygen in the baby. Delivery of the baby is the best cure for preeclampsia. If preeclampsia becomes life-threatening to the mother or baby and the baby must be delivered before its due date, there is a greater risk that the baby will have breathing problems and be underweight.

As for your overall life expectancy, there is no evidence that pregnancy shortens the lives of women with diabetes. The only exception is if you have established coronary artery disease, in which case your physician will probably recommend that you avoid pregnancy altogether.

Possible Risks to the Baby

The effects of your diabetes on your unborn baby depend on your blood sugar control during pregnancy: the better the diabetes control, the fewer the complications. High blood sugar levels in the mother during the critical early weeks of pregnancy greatly increase the risk that the baby will be born with birth defects. The babies of women with very poor diabetes control (measured as high glycosylated hemoglobin) during the first three months of pregnancy have a 20 to 25 percent chance of having birth defects. This compares to 2 to 3 percent for the general population, as well as for women with well-controlled diabetes from before conception through the entire pregnancy.

Later in pregnancy, high blood sugar levels in the mother are passed on to the fetus, stimulating the baby to produce too much insulin and grow unusually large. Sometimes the baby grows too large to pass through the birth canal, and a cesarean delivery is performed. High insulin levels may also prevent the unborn baby's lungs and other organs from maturing at a normal pace. After birth, the baby may have severe hypoglycemia when it no longer receives glucose from its mother but it is still making large amounts of insulin. High blood glucose levels in the mother are also associated with unexplained fetal death late in pregnancy.

Will your baby develop diabetes later in life? If you have insulin-dependent diabetes, the chances that your child will one day develop diabetes are low—about 2 percent during the first twenty years of life. If you have non-insulin-dependent diabetes, the risk that your child will develop diabetes as an adult is considerably higher, the exact figure depending on whether he or she becomes obese and the intensity of your and the father's family history of diabetes.

How to Reduce the Risks to You and Your Baby

As you have probably guessed by now, the best way to prevent most of the diabetes-related complications of pregnancy and to ensure a healthy baby is control, control, control! Here's a look at what you can expect from your health team, and what will be expected of you during pregnancy.

Your Pregnancy Health Care Team

Pregnancy is a special time for all women. For the woman with diabetes, it is also a good time to seek out the care of a team of highly trained medical specialists. The ideal treatment team should include an internist interested in the treatment of diabetes during pregnancy, an obstetrician with experience in the treatment of pregnancies complicated by diabetes, a certified diabetes educator, a nutritionist familiar with the needs of both pregnancy and diabetes, and a pediatrician for the baby when it is born. A hospital with a specialized high-risk pregnancy team and sophisticated equipment should be chosen when the possibility of complications exists. If you don't have easy access to such a medical center, you should at least see a physician who has a particular interest in managing pregnancy complicated by diabetes. If you don't know of one, ask your regular doctor, other mothers with diabetes, or your local affiliate of the American Diabetes Association (address on page 187).

In the early part of your pregnancy, you will probably see your internist once a week. You should also be examined by your obstetrician as soon as you discover that you are pregnant, and every three or four weeks thereafter. By the end of the second trimester, you will be seeing your obstetrician once a week and will probably maintain daily telephone contact with your internist to keep up with your changing insulin needs.

Prepregnancy Care

Ideally, if you are a woman with diabetes, prenatal care should begin with a visit to your doctor *before you conceive*. At this preconception visit, your doctor can measure your blood pressure, check your eyes, check the health of your heart with an electrocardiogram (ECG), perform urine tests to determine whether you have kidney problems, and check your overall diabetes control with a glycosylated hemoglobin test. Your physician may also have you undergo a blood test to see whether you have already been exposed to rubella (German measles), which can cause severe birth defects if the mother contracts rubella during early pregnancy, whether or not she has diabetes. Undergoing these tests before you conceive can help prevent any diabetes-related complications from worsening during pregnancy—you may need laser photocoagulation treatment for proliferative diabetic retinopathy, for instance. If your diabetes is not well controlled, you and your physician can work toward achieving better control before you conceive. And if you haven't been exposed to rubella and have no natural immunity, your doctor may recommend that you be vaccinated before you get pregnant. If you have non-insulin-dependent diabetes and take oral medication to control it, your doctor will probably have you switch to insulin at this time, since it is not known what effect diabetes pills have on the developing fetus.

This is also a good time to meet with your nutrition counselor to discuss your increased nutritional needs during pregnancy. You should also review your exercise program with your doctor. (If you don't already exercise regularly, you may want to start now—*before* you get pregnant. Talk to your doctor, and see Chapter 4 for details.) If you smoke cigarettes or drink alcohol, now is the time to quit. These substances, even when used in moderation, can harm the growing fetus and are strictly off limits during pregnancy.

If your blood sugar levels are not very stable, you should use some form of contraception until diabetes control improves. Remember: the danger of birth defects is much greater for babies whose mothers had poor diabetes control in the first two to three months of pregnancy. This includes the time before you know you're pregnant, which is why good control is essential before you get pregnant.

When You Become Pregnant

When your blood glucose levels are as near normal as possible, your doctor will tell you when it's safe to stop using contraception. Even if you are not sure you're pregnant while you are actively trying to conceive, you should control your diabetes as though you were already pregnant.

Once you conceive, you'll need to work hard to keep blood glucose levels near normal throughout your pregnancy. If you take insulin, your physician will tailor an insulin schedule to your needs. Most women who take insulin will require at least two injections daily, and some may need up to four injections a day. If you used an insulin pump before you got pregnant, you can continue using it throughout your pregnancy, if you wish. You should know, however, that the insulin pump has no particular advantage over multiple injections during pregnancy, and it may have some *disadvantages*, particularly if the pump breaks down or the needle site gets infected.

A key to good diabetes control during pregnancy is regular self-monitoring of your blood sugar levels. Ask your doctor how often you should test. Generally speaking, women who take insulin will need to test their blood sugar levels before each meal and possibly one to two hours after eating. If you have hypoglycemic symptoms in the middle of the night, have persistent low blood sugar or elevated blood sugar first thing in the morning, or are using an insulin pump, your physician may recommend that you also test your blood sugar at 2:00 or 3:00 A.M. from time to time. Throughout your pregnancy, you should write down your glucose values in a diabetes diary, along with comments about your calorie intake and exercise activity. You will also be instructed to test your urine for ketones before breakfast every day and any time blood glucose levels exceed 200 mg/dl. In addition, your physician will perform a glycosylated hemoglobin test at your first prenatal visit and at least once every three months throughout your pregnancy.

Overall, if your diabetes was well controlled *before* you got pregnant, you probably will have very few problems during your pregnancy. If the diabetes has not been well controlled, you may have more trouble getting it under control before conception and during pregnancy, but with a team effort, it can be done. Be sure to keep glucagon on hand and make certain that family and friends know how to give an injection. (See page 108) Fortunately, there is no evidence that the baby is harmed by the mother's occasional hypoglycemic spells.

Eating for Two When You Have Diabetes

Even though you are "eating for two" now, your calorie intake *doesn't* double. Your nutrition counselor will work with you to adjust your meal plan to meet your increased caloric needs. Generally speaking, you'll need to eat about a third more calories during pregnancy than you did before you conceived. If you are overweight when you conceive or gain weight too rapidly in the early part of your pregnancy, your nutrition counselor will probably adjust your calorie intake accordingly. *Don't* try to cut back on calories on your own during pregnancy. The baby's normal growth and development depend on adequate calories from the mother. Pregnancy is *not* the time to go on a weight-reducing diet. You should plan to eat sensibly *and* gain weight (most women gain twenty to twenty-five pounds) during your pregnancy.

Your nutrition counselor will probably recommend that you eat about 10 percent of your daily calories as a light breakfast, 30 percent at lunch, and 30 percent at supper. The remaining 30 percent of calories should be distributed among several snacks. You'll need a bedtime snack to decrease the risk of nighttime hypoglycemia.

As for *what* you should eat, you should rely on the same healthy eating habits during pregnancy that you normally use to help keep your diabetes in check. (See Chapter 3.) Talk with your nutrition counselor about ways to handle morning sickness and food cravings, especially if you crave foods that aren't a major part of your meal plan, like pickles (high salt) and ice cream (high fat). Alternative sweeteners such as Nutrasweet are okay to use during pregnancy.

What About Exercise?

Although there isn't enough scientific data to make specific recommendations about exercise during pregnancy if you have diabetes, it is probably all right to continue your regular exercise program during your pregnancy, provided you have your doctor's approval, you don't find it too taxing, and you don't experience hypoglycemia as a result. Brisk walking is an excellent activity during pregnancy. Pregnancy is *not* a good time to begin a vigorous exercise program.

Prenatal Tests

Because women with diabetes do run a greater risk of developing certain pregnancy-related complications, your doctor will recommend that you undergo a number of prenatal screening tests, including the following:

Maternal serum alpha-fetoprotein. Alpha-fetoprotein (AFP) is a protein produced by the fetus. High levels in the mother's blood may indicate the presence of a congenital abnormality, such as a neural tube defect (an abnormality of the brain and spinal cord tissues in the fetus). Extremely low levels of AFP in the mother's blood suggest there may be a chromosomal abnormality, such as Down syndrome. (Chromosomal abnormalities, such as Down syndrome, do not occur more often in babies of mothers with diabetes.) The test is usually performed between the 14th and 20th weeks of pregnancy.

Ultrasound. This is a test in which sound waves are used to create an image of your baby on a video screen. Ultrasound can detect some physical deformities in midpregnancy, including neural tube and heart defects, cleft palate, and problems with the abdominal wall, stomach, kidneys, and bladder. This painless procedure takes fifteen to twenty minutes. While you are lying on your back on an examining table, an ultrasound technician spreads an oil or gel over your abdomen and moves a hand-held ultrasound transmitter slowly across it. In the last months of your pregnancy, your doctor may use ultrasound to determine the size of the baby, its activity, its breathing movements, and other signs of well-being.

Amniocentesis. In this test, a sample of the fluid in the birth sac is taken through a long needle inserted through the abdomen and into the amniotic sac. Because both fluid and cells from the fetus are in the sample, it can be used to check for a number of birth defects, including the chromosomal abnormality Down syndrome, around the twentieth week of your pregnancy. The test is also used in late pregnancy to check the maturity of the baby's lungs, which is important if your baby is likely to be premature.

Fetal echocardiography. The structure of the baby's heart is determined by this test, which also uses ultrasound.

Nonstress test. Usually performed in your doctor's office, the nonstress test involves having your doctor record the baby's heart rate with a fetal monitor attached to two elasticized belts that are strapped comfortably around your abdomen. Your doctor will look for characteristic changes in the baby's heart rate that are signs of the baby's well-being.

Self-monitoring of fetal activity. In addition to the nonstress test, you will probably be instructed to monitor your baby's activity in the womb daily after the twenty-eighth week of pregnancy. This involves lying down on your left side once a day and counting your baby's movements. Once the baby has moved ten times, you can stop counting. If the baby does not move ten times in two hours you should promptly call your obstetrician, who will want to examine you and possibly perform a nonstress test.

Most women with diabetes can safely manage their pregnancy *and* their diabetes without hospitalization. If you have kidney disease or hypertension, if your diabetes is poorly controlled, or if the baby is in jeopardy, hospitalization may be necessary to regulate the diabetes or monitor your condition and the baby's.

Labor and Delivery

In the past, babies of women with diabetes were delivered before or during the thirty-seventh week of pregnancy to reduce the risk of fetal death. Today, however, doctors have a variety of tests to monitor the baby more closely during the final weeks of pregnancy. This allows the fetus to remain in the safety of the mother's womb as long as possible. Premature delivery of a baby is associated with respiratory problems and low birth weight; the longer the baby stays in the womb, the less likely it is to develop these problems.

When your due date arrives, your physician may decide to induce labor if it hasn't already begun. If you take insulin, you will probably receive insulin intravenously during active labor, or during the operation if you have a cesarean delivery. Hourly blood glucose measurements will be taken to ensure that you don't have hypoglycemia. After the baby is born, your physician will help you adjust your insulin dosage as needed for the change in your metabolism.

If you have diabetes-related problems with your heart or circulatory system, if your diabetes is poorly controlled, if you have had a previous stillbirth, or if you have not received regular prenatal care, your doctor may decide to deliver the baby early—usually around the thirty-eighth week of pregnancy. Before the baby is delivered, the health care team will perform an amniocentesis to see whether the baby's lungs have matured enough for normal breathing. If the baby's lungs are still immature at thirty-eight weeks, the delivery may be postponed, provided the baby shows no signs of distress.

If You Have Gestational Diabetes

Nine out of ten pregnant women with diabetes have *gestational diabetes*, a form of diabetes that occurs only during pregnancy and disappears after the baby is born. Because gestational diabetes doesn't develop until the second half of pregnancy, women with this form of diabetes do not have a greater chance of having a baby with birth defects than women without diabetes. If the diabetes is not controlled, however, the baby may get excess glucose from the mother, forcing it to produce excess insulin and become too large for its degree of maturity, and the baby may have to be delivered by cesarean section.

Prenatal care of the woman with gestational diabetes is similar to that for the woman who had diabetes before pregnancy. Often, mild cases of gestational diabetes can be managed with good eating habits alone. Women with more severe diabetes may need to take insulin as well.

If you develop gestational diabetes, your body should return to normal after you deliver the baby. Many women with gestational diabetes, however, are at a greater risk of developing diabetes later in life. By keeping up the good eating and exercise habits you learned during your pregnancy, you will substantially reduce your odds of developing diabetes in the years to come.

* * *

Pregnancy is a time of great excitement and apprehension for *all* women. If you have diabetes, you may be even more excited about the possibility of having a baby (particularly if you were under the impression that you couldn't or shouldn't have children)—and more apprehensive about the possible risks.

No amount of reassurance can ease *all* of your anxieties, but by receiving excellent care before and during your pregnancy and doing everything you can to keep your diabetes under control, you'll dramatically increase your odds of having a complication-free pregnancy and delivering a healthy baby.

CHAPTER 10

Special Needs

When you have diabetes, the stress of illness, surgery, or travel can trigger significant changes in blood sugar levels, as can everyday emotional stress. With a little advance preparation, however, you can avert any dangerous changes in glucose levels that could lead to complications.

Preparing for an Unexpected Illness

A cold, the flu, a fever, or even an infected cut or sore can cause blood sugar levels to rise. Taking extra steps to control your diabetes when you are ill can keep a minor problem from escalating into something more serious.

Your doctor or diabetes educator will advise you about a plan for your sick days. They will include in this plan how to monitor your blood for glucose and (if you have insulin-dependent diabetes) your urine for ketones, which over-the-counter medications you should have on hand, and how you should modify your diet. Here are some general recommendations:

1. Keep your medicine cabinet stocked with a fever thermometer, aspirin or other pain relievers, a liquid antacid for heartburn or stomachaches, an antidiarrheal medication, and rectal suppositories for vomiting. Ask your doctor whether you should keep a short-acting insulin on hand if you do not usually use one. If you take oral hypoglycemic drugs, you should be aware that many drugs interact with these medications. (See page 72.) Be sure to check with your doctor before taking any other medication.

2. Consider ahead of time what you might be able to eat when you are feeling too sick to make decisions. Review the "Guidelines for Eating When You Are Ill" (below) with your diabetes educator or physician and incorporate some of your favorite foods.

3. Familiarize yourself with some common signs and symptoms of infection. These include fever, bleeding gums, swollen tender lymph nodes in the neck or groin, burning and pain on urination, and vaginal itching.

4. If you have signs of infection or illness, monitor your glucose levels *every four hours.*

5. If you have insulin-dependent diabetes, check your urine for ketones *every four hours.* Contact your doctor immediately if you discover ketones in your urine.

6. Continue your current diabetes medication schedule even if you are not eating. You usually need *more* insulin, not less, when you are sick. Many people with diabetes are hospitalized during illnesses because they didn't take their oral medication or insulin. *Avoid this mistake.*

7. Know when to call the doctor. As a rule, you should contact your physician when

- you realize you have an infection or illness
- you have consistently high or low blood glucose levels
- there are ketones in your urine
- you can't keep food or liquids down, for more than four hours
- you are unable to eat normally, for more than twelve hours
- you are breathing faster or deeper than normal
- you have a fever
- you have headache, confusion, or weakness and fatigue

When you call or someone calls for you, be prepared to report temperature, blood glucose test results, urine test results for ketones, eating patterns, any vomiting or diarrhea, or signs of infection or illness. If your doctor can't be reached, go to the emergency room of your local hospital.

Guidelines for Eating When You Are Ill

Understandably, you may not feel like eating much when you are ill. But you need food and fluids to recover. The guidelines here are based on your symptoms and how much food you can tolerate. For instance, if you are having trouble keeping food down, don't force yourself to eat solid foods. Instead, sip the fluids listed in Stage 1 and gradually progress to the next stage as your symptoms improve. If you can tolerate most foods, start with the bland diet in Stage 4 until you feel well enough to resume your regular diet.

STAGE 1

Symptoms: Severe nausea, vomiting, severe diarrhea, fever.
Foods: Orange juice, grapefruit juice, tomato juice, soup,

broth, coffee, tea, regular soft drinks (shake out the carbonation).

Frequency: Sip a tablespoonful of liquid every ten to fifteen minutes.

Note: If you can't keep down liquids at this frequency, be sure to call your doctor. Advance to the next stage when the nausea and vomiting have almost stopped.

STAGE 2

Symptoms: Little or no appetite, occasional diarrhea, fatigue, fever.

Foods: Cream soup, mashed potatoes, cooked cereal, plain yogurt, banana, ice cream, fruit-flavored gelatins, juice, broth, regular soft drinks.

Frequency: Take ½ cup to 1 cup of food or liquid every one or two hours.

Note: When you have a fever, you perspire and lose body fluids. In addition to the above foods, be sure to drink water or a light beverage every ten to fifteen minutes. Move to Stage 3 when you have had several servings from this stage and your symptoms are improving.

STAGE 3

Symptoms: Limited appetite but can eat small meals, slight fever, can sit up or walk, still sluggish.

Foods: You can now select foods from your regular food plan if they agree with you. You don't, however, have to eat your protein and fat food choices. You might want to change your usual menu to foods more appetizing to you.

Milk serving: Instead of one cup of milk, try:
Cream soup   (1 cup)
Plain yogurt   (1 cup)

Sweetened custard   (½ cup; omit one fruit
                                     serving)

Bread and cereal serving: You can eat one of these foods
as your usual bread or starch serving:

Bread   (1 slice)
Cooked cereal   (½ cup)
Mashed potatoes   (½ cup)
Saltines   (6 squares)
Vanilla wafers   (6)
Soup—noodle or starchy   (1 cup)
Ice cream   (½ cup)
Sherbet   (¼ cup)
Fruit-flavored gelatin   (½ cup)
Regular soft drinks   (¾ cup)

Vegetable serving: You can eat ½ serving from the bread
and cereal list above.

Fruit serving: You can eat one of these foods instead of
your usual fruit serving:

Unsweetened applesauce   (½ cup)
Apple, grape, prune juice   (⅓ cup)
Orange or grapefruit   (½ cup)
   juice
Banana   (½)
Popsicle   (½)
Regular soft drinks   (½ cup)

Frequency: Eat as many meals and snacks as you usually do,
according to your meal plan. Usually this means three
meals and an evening snack.

Note: Some of the foods listed here (such as regular soft
drinks) are high in sugar and would not be regularly used
when you are not sick. Move on to Stage 4 when you have
had several meals at this stage and are having no problems
with nausea or digestion. If you still have a fever, remember to drink several extra glasses of water, weak tea, or a
diet soft drink every day.

STAGE 4

Symptoms: Still feeling generally sick; heavy or spicy foods cause stomach upset.

Foods: Continue with your regular plan, avoiding spicy or high-fat foods. For your protein serving, choose foods mild in taste and easy to digest, such as scrambled or soft-boiled eggs, cottage cheese, broiled fish, or baked chicken without heavy sauces. Eat your fruit, vegetables, starch, and protein in moderate amounts according to your usual meal plan.

Frequency: Eat at regular meal and snack times.

Note: Move back to your regular plan if you have no problem with these foods for a day. If you feel worse, drop back a stage for a day or until you feel better.

Having Surgery

The physical stress of surgery and postoperative pain can raise blood glucose levels. Thanks to advances in the methods of controlling blood sugar during an operation, this is no longer a serious problem, and most people with diabetes can now undergo surgery with little more than the normal risks associated with an operation. The only difference: your blood sugar levels will be carefully monitored before, during, and after the surgery to reduce the risks of hyperglycemia, hypoglycemia, and ketoacidosis associated with an operation.

Elective Surgery

Unless you are having emergency surgery, your physician will want you to achieve optimum control of your blood sugar levels before entering the hospital. To prepare yourself for surgery, try to get into the best physical shape possible through diet and exercise. Before surgery, you can also expect to undergo a full physical exam to ensure that you are not suffering from any diabetes-related complications, such as kidney or heart disease. Your doctor may recommend that you monitor your blood sugar levels more diligently on the days just before your operation to ensure that your diabetes is under control. If your diabetes control has been poor, you may need to enter the hospital a few days early so that the staff can monitor and adjust your glucose and insulin levels more precisely.

Once you are in the hospital, your health care team will take charge of your diabetes management. If you have non-insulin-dependent diabetes that is controlled without medication, you will be treated in the same way as people who don't have diabetes, with one exception: your blood glucose levels will be monitored more closely after surgery. This is because hyperglycemia can result from the stress of surgery and postoperative discomfort. Most of the time, this postoperative rise in blood sugar levels is only temporary. If blood glucose levels higher than 250 mg/dl persist, you may receive small doses of insulin.

If you take oral diabetes medication or insulin and you are having major surgery under general anesthesia, you will continue your regular medication plan until the morning of surgery. Then one or two intravenous feeding lines will be placed in your arm or hand so that glucose and insulin can flow directly into your bloodstream. This gives your physician better control over glucose or insulin delivery. Throughout the operation, your anesthesiologist will measure Your blood sugar concentrations hourly with a glucose meter and give you insulin or glucose as needed.

When you wake up, nurses will continue to monitor your glucose levels in the recovery room and on the ward. You will continue receiving insulin intravenously until you are strong enough to eat. At this point, you will switch back to your regular insulin or oral medication regimen. Your glucose levels will continue to be checked regularly.

If you are having minor outpatient surgery without general anesthesia and expect to eat the same day, your physician may have you delay your usual medication and eating schedule until after surgery. As soon as you can eat, you will receive your oral medication. If you have insulin-dependent diabetes, you will probably receive your insulin injection on time, although the dose may be reduced, even if you don't eat until after surgery. In either case, your physician will expect you or family members to continue to monitor your glucose levels when you get home.

Dental Surgery

People with diabetes are more prone to developing dental infections and periodontal disease (an advanced form of gum disease), and these problems often require extensive dental procedures that make it difficult to eat. When you have dental surgery, you will probably miss at least one meal, which will affect your blood sugar levels. If you take insulin or oral medication and are having extensive dental work done, be sure to work out your medication and eating schedule with your physician and dentist beforehand. Try to schedule your appointment for first thing in the morning so that you will miss as few meals as possible.

If you take oral medications and expect to miss one meal, you will probably be advised to skip your morning dosage and resume your regular regimen once you begin eating again. If you take a long-acting drug such as chlorpropamide (Diabinese), you may be advised to stop taking it the day before your dental appointment.

If you take insulin, your physician may lower your dosage if you expect to miss a meal. Even if you miss a meal, you still need some insulin, as the stress of the procedure or the presence of a gum infection may cause glucose levels to rise. You should monitor your glucose level much more closely before and after the procedure. Be sure to discuss all necessary steps with your physician.

Traveling with Diabetes

Vacations and travel provide a welcome break from routine. But traveling—particularly through several time zones—often involves changes in your eating, your level of physical activity, your sleep schedule, and your stress level, all of which can affect your blood sugar levels. You'll need to do a little advanced planning and take a few extra precautions while you travel, particularly if you are insulin-dependent. Here are some travel tips to ensure that when you go on vacation, control of your diabetes doesn't take a vacation, too:

• If you take insulin, consult with your physician or diabetes educator before you leave. You may need to adjust the timing of your meals and the amount or timing of your insulin dose, particularly if your travel takes you across several time zones.

• While traveling, plan to test your blood glucose more frequently than you would at home.

• If you are traveling with others, have your travel companions carry an extra set of supplies for you and make sure they know how to help you in an emergency.

• Always carry a wallet card or medical bracelet indicating that you have diabetes.

• Keep your medication, insulin, and syringes readily available at all times in your carry-on luggage. You should also bring along a letter signed by your doctor explaining why you are carrying these supplies. (For more on what and how to pack, see "Packing Your Bags," page 165.)

• Find out in advance how and where to obtain emergency medical help at your destination. If you are traveling abroad, you can obtain a list of diabetes associations in the countries you plan to visit, as well as information on local food customs and the availability of medical assistance and insulin by writing to the American Diabetes Association (see page 187 for address); the International Diabetes Federation (IDF), 10 Queen Street, London, W1M OBD, England; IDF at the International Association Center, 40 Washington Street, 1050 Brussels, Belgium; or Intermedic, 777 Third Avenue, New York, NY 10017 (phone: 212/486-8976). For a list of English-speaking physicians in the countries you are visiting (as well as information on the climate, food, and sanitary conditions), write to the International Association for Medical Assistance to Travelers, 417 Center Street, Lewiston, NY 14092. The doctors on the list have agreed to treat anyone who is a member of this organization (membership requires only a token donation).

• If you are traveling abroad, be sure to get any immunizations you need at least one month before your trip. Sometimes immunizations can cause a reaction and throw off your diabetes control, so it's best to get your immunizations while you are still under your own doctor's supervision. (For information on immunizations, contact your local health department.)

• If you plan to visit a non-English-speaking country, you may want to learn a few phrases in the country's language, such as "I have diabetes," "I need a doctor," or

"Sugar or fruit juice, please." Your local librarian or a foreign language teacher at a nearby school may be able to help you find materials. Write these phrases on a note card and carry it with you at all times.

• If you must purchase insulin in another country, remember that variations in refinement, purity, strength, brand, type, species, or method of manufacture may result in the need for a change in dosage. Keep in mind, too, that U-100 insulin may not be available. If this is the case, buy syringes to match the insulin (probably U-40 or U-80) and give yourself *the same number of units as usual*. Do not try to calculate how much U-40 solution you should use in a U-100 syringe.

• If you need to purchase oral medication, make sure you know the generic (chemical) name for your drug, since brand names may differ in foreign countries.

• When traveling by air, drink plenty of fluids. The air in the airline cabin is extremely dry, making it possible to become dehydrated without realizing it. Before boarding the plane, drink one 8-ounce glass of a nonalcoholic beverage for a short (2–3 hour) flight and 2–3 glasses for longer flights. Drink another glass of fluid each hour you are in the air. (Avoid alcoholic beverages, which also cause dehydration.)

• While traveling, try to eat at least every four hours. If you are traveling by air, you may want to call the airline (more than twenty-four hours ahead of flight departure) and request a special meal to match your diabetes meal plan. (You should also pack your own meal in case your special meal doesn't make it onto the plane, or in case the airline doesn't serve food on your flight.) If you are traveling with a child who has diabetes, remember that the child may need more calories than usual, so bring along extra meals and snacks.

• If your activity level is greater than normal while you are on vacation, have an extra snack between meals.

• No matter what kind of transportation you use, get up and walk around every two hours. Sitting still for long periods may elevate your blood sugar levels and can induce urinary infection. Walking helps combat travel fatigue, improves your circulation, and helps keep blood glucose levels on a more even keel.

Packing Your Bags

You should always keep the following supplies on hand in a carry-on bag:

• your usual supply of oral medication or insulin, syringes, and materials to test for glucose and ketones.
• a *backup supply* (at least a week's supply or preferably a duplicate of your regular supply) of insulin, syringes, and testing materials. *Always take more than you need* in case you are delayed somewhere or break an insulin bottle.
• a glucagon emergency kit (if you take insulin).
• a container for disposing of your syringes. (A small empty plastic soda bottle works nicely.)
• any other travel medications you may need (such as motion sickness pills, medication for vomiting, diarrhea, or constipation, and an antibiotic ointment) that have already been approved by your doctor.
• easy-to-carry snacks, such as cheese or peanut butter and crackers, granola, or trail mix. In addition, bring a quick-acting glucose preparation, such as glucose tablets

or hard candies, in case you have a hypoglycemic episode.
- Extra food, especially if you expect to be traveling in countries where food availability is unpredictable.
- a doctor's written prescription for your medications and syringes.
- a note explaining why you carry insulin and syringes, to avoid problems with security or customs.
- an identification card or bracelet stating that you have diabetes.

When packing your travel kit, check all the lids of your medications and insulin to make sure they are on tight. Keep your insulin or oral medications in their original packages or in smaller packages that are clearly marked with the generic (chemical) name, strength, and dosage; this helps avoid confusion if you have to refill your prescriptions in a foreign country. To protect your insulin from extreme temperatures and breakage, try packing it in a short wide-mouthed insulated bottle or jug: fill the jug with cold water or ice to lower the internal temperature; place your insulin vials in a plastic bag, wrap the bag in a cool, wet washcloth, then empty the jug and place the entire package in the jug. Insulated insulin travel bags and cold packs are also available. Check your pharmacy.

In your checked luggage, be sure to pack a sunscreen and clothing to protect you from the sun, such as a lightweight jacket or long-sleeved shirts, and a hat. Severe sunburn can lead to changes in blood sugar levels and is bad for your skin. Comfortable walking shoes will protect your feet from cuts, infections, and blisters. (*Never* walk barefoot outdoors.) Be sure to break in your shoes before leaving, and bring two pairs. Bring enough socks or stockings so that you can change them every day. Remember, an infection can lead to a rise in blood sugar. Bring moleskin to apply to places on your feet that start to turn red. Pack any extra insulin in plastic bags between layers of clothing in your suitcase. This helps guard against breakage and exposure to extreme temperatures.

When you reach your destination, refrigerate your insulin as soon as possible and lock up your syringes—in either your carry-on bag or suitcase. Dispose of your syringe and needle properly, as you learned at home.

Coping with Everyday Stress

Even the stresses of everyday life can affect your blood sugar levels. Stress is an inevitable and a necessary part of life. After all, a roller coaster ride or a horror movie wouldn't be the same if it didn't make your heart pound. A racing heart and other physical changes also take place when the stress is less pleasurable: being stuck in rush-hour traffic, having an argument with your spouse or partner, or even solving a simple arithmetic problem. Less noticeable chemical changes occur in your body in the face of major long-term stresses, such as losing a loved one or coping with a family member's illness. But even such "positive" stresses as moving to a new town, getting a promotion, or making new friends can affect your body chemistry.

This physical reaction to emotional or mental stress is an inborn survival trait known as the "fight or flight response," which developed when prehistoric people had to contend with such physical threats as wild animals. And while the source of stress has changed over the years, your body's basic reaction hasn't: your adrenal glands (two small glands situated just above the kidneys) begin churning out the "stress" hormones *epinephrine* (sometimes called *adrenaline)* and *norepinephrine*, priming your body for action. These hormones accelerate your breathing and pulse rate, raise your blood pressure, and release stored sugars from the liver into the bloodstream, providing your body with quick energy—and raising your blood sugar levels.

These stress-related increases in blood sugar levels may upset the balance you are trying to achieve through diet, exercise, and medication. To restore that balance, you will either have to change the way you respond to stress or adjust your diet, exercise, and medication accordingly.

How will you know when you are under "too much stress"? As you are probably aware, when your blood sugar rises significantly, your body will give you warning signs that something is wrong. You may feel thirsty, need to urinate more often, feel weak, or have stomach pain, nausea, or vomiting. Your vision may become blurry. Call your physician if any of these symptoms persist.

You should also monitor your blood glucose levels more often during times of stress. If you take insulin, check your urine for ketones if your blood sugar is greater than 240 mg/dl. Call your doctor if ketones are present, as you will require more insulin than you usually take.

Living with stress is obviously a challenge, as stress affects each of us every day. To combat the physical problems that arise when you feel stressed, try to establish preventive coping methods so that blood glucose levels don't rise needlessly. Here are a few ideas:

Exercise regularly. Exercise is one of the most effective methods you have of alleviating stress. Exercise reduces muscle tension and helps put the stress hormones to their intended use, making you feel more relaxed. If you exercise regularly, you will have more energy and a lower anxiety level and will be more prepared to deal with the problems you face daily. See Chapter 4 and talk with your diabetes educator about setting up an exercise program tailored to your needs.

Make time for yourself. As a part of your daily plan, set aside time to exercise or work on a favorite hobby or activity. Taking time for yourself allows you to relax and maintain a clearer picture of the world around you. You may feel less governed by events and more in control of your life.

Practice relaxation exercises. There are many relaxation training programs, such as yoga, progressive relaxation, and biofeedback, that teach stretching, breathing, and meditation to increase a sense of calm and well-being. When you are feeling more centered, you are less likely to react strongly or to be bothered by minor incidents. Strong emotional reactions are draining and can adversely affect your blood glucose levels.

Think positively. If you try to approach the day positively, thinking of what you *can* do instead of what you *can't*, you will tend to feel more upbeat and in control. You'll be more prepared to meet the unexpected, and therefore will tend to feel more relaxed and less stressed.

Set priorities. Do you always expect to accomplish more than is humanly possible? Do you race through the day with a feeling of pressure that you will never accomplish what *must* be done? Try to evaluate your goals for the day honestly. Set priorities and reasonable expectations. Avoid the rush through traffic by leaving work five or ten minutes early or fifteen minutes late. Make time allowances that let you get to where you want to go on time without the hurry. Try not to be the super-mom, -dad or -friend who must be everywhere at once, all things to all people. Think about what you consider important and set out to accomplish what is manageable.

Talk it out. Communicating with family, friends, or even a professional counselor can also provide relief from stress, as expressing emotions tends to leave you feeling unburdened. Avoid letting your feelings build up to the point of explosion. This can take an enormous toll on your emotional and physical health.

Having diabetes, of course, is stressful in itself. Consider contacting a diabetes support group in your area. (See page 187 for a referral to diabetes support groups in your area.)

Often just talking about the difficulties you face every day and discovering you are not alone in your struggle can be comforting and can relieve tension or frustration. Some diabetes groups might even have lists of members to call, so that you can regularly talk with people who understand exactly how you feel.

CHAPTER 11

When a Child Has Diabetes

On top of the normal developmental issues that all parents and children face—a toddler's temper tantrums, an adolescent's assertions of independence and vulnerability to peer pressure—as parents of a child with diabetes, you will also have to deal with the burden of diabetes.

As a parent, you will play a central role in your child's diabetes management and care plan, a role that will change as your child grows. Here are some of the most common age-related issues.

The Early Years

When a young child is diagnosed with diabetes, you, the parents, will have to perform virtually all of the day-to-day care responsibilities yourselves, including meal planning and preparation, giving insulin injections, monitoring, and record-keeping. All of this may seem overwhelming at first, but as the weeks progress, you will quickly gain confidence. It helps if you can divide up the caretaking responsibilities between two adults in the home (for example, father and mother, mother and grandmother, father and grown-up sister) so that neither feels overly burdened and resentful. Maintaining regular contact with your child's medical team, including the doctor and diabetes educator, can help you cope as well. You may also want to seek out the support of other parents of children with diabetes.

During the early childhood years, one of the biggest problems you may face is being able to tell the difference between normal behavior, such as an infant's distress or a toddler's temper tantrums, and a hypoglycemic episode. To complicate matters, children in this age group are often finicky eaters, so they have a greater tendency to develop low blood sugar reactions. For these reasons, frequent monitoring of your child's blood sugar levels is essential. If your child is a picky eater, offer a wide variety of nutritious foods at snacktimes and mealtimes, and let your child choose. Whatever you do, remain calm and try not to make an issue out of eating or make the dinner table a battleground.

Toddlers and preschoolers may balk at taking insulin injections or having their blood tested, throwing temper tantrums or hiding. Preschoolers may even view your attempts to manage their diabetes as a form of punishment. Take a matter-of-fact approach, and give plenty of hugs and kisses both before and after the injection or blood test. It often helps to give the toddler some measure of control by letting him or her choose which finger to stick or which injection site to use. Sometimes letting the toddler pretend to give insulin injections to a doll helps ease anxiety.

School-Age and Preadolescent Children (Five to Eleven Years)

Younger children often think of diabetes as a punishment for something bad that they have done. At seven or eight years of age, going to a diabetes camp (either a day camp or a residential one) can be very helpful in working through these feelings.

Going to school means having to trust others to recognize the symptoms of hypoglycemia, which requires good communication with the school personnel. Plan to spend some time with your child's teacher and the school's administrators, making sure they know how to recognize and cope with insulin reactions, as well as whom to contact and what to do in an emergency. Don't allow the school to deal inappropriately with your child's diabetes by recommending home teaching so that school personnel don't have to worry about it. If school administrators or teachers make such recommendations, talk to your diabetes care team about educating these professionals about diabetes.

At this age, children may begin to try using the diabetes as an excuse to get out of going to school. Diabetes is not an excuse for getting out of physical education or missing extracurricular activities. Arrangements can always be made for testing, if it needs to be done during school, or snacking, and the treatment team can help develop any special schedules and permissions necessary.

One of your goals as your child gets older and can understand more is to increase his or her responsibility for diabetes care consistent with his or her ability. A good way to determine whether your child is ready to take on more responsibility is to have him or her teach a particular aspect of diabetes control to somebody else—yourself, a brother or sister, a friend, or a teacher. Once your child has a solid understanding of the task at hand, as well as the motor skills and coordination to do it, you can start making a gradual transition, fully supervising your child at first and slowly easing up on your supervision over weeks or months. Give plenty of praise and reassurance for a job well done, and *never* scold or punish your child for poor performance. Be prepared to step in again if your child becomes ill or for some reason or another slips up in his or her diabetes care.

It is also a good idea to let older children in this age group (eight- to eleven-year-olds) talk directly to the health team members from time to time to learn how to make decisions about their diabetes care.

Adolescence

The hormonal changes and growth spurts that occur during puberty naturally affect your child's insulin dosages and dietary needs. These physical changes often require more supervision by you and your child's health team in making adjustments in insulin dosages and diet. Unfortunately, these normal physical changes occur at a time when the psychological changes of adolescence—notably a need for more independence and a tendency to rebel—are also making themselves known. Obviously, if your teenager rebels against his or her diabetes care plan by skipping meals, eating mostly junk food, taking insulin at the wrong time or not at all, refusing to monitor blood sugar levels, or making up test results, diabetes control will suffer.

Most teenagers are not willing to let you control their diabetes, but most are incapable of or unwilling to care for themselves totally. In spite of these problems, teenagers with diabetes manage to survive these tumultuous years. With a little understanding and a *lot* of patience, you can, too. Here are a few tips to follow:

• Be willing to compromise on some aspects of your child's diabetes care plan. Talk with your child's doctor (or have your child do so) about areas of your child's diabetes care plan in which there is room for negotiation and compromise. Although insulin injections are usually *nonnegotiable*, you may be able to negotiate other aspects of the diabetes care plan, such as the times and frequency of blood glucose testing.

• Try to keep issues related to diabetes and those related to normal development separate. For instance, when setting a curfew, don't say, "You can't stay out late because it will interfere with your diabetes control." Instead, explain that your child can't stay out late because he or she is too young.

• Consider diabetes camp. Teenagers are extremely concerned about their self-image and about not being different. Having diabetes can make them feel different because they constantly have to watch what they eat, monitor their blood, take insulin, and guard against insulin reactions. Even a teenager who has had diabetes since early childhood and who seems to have adjusted well may suddenly feel he or she doesn't fit in. Teen support groups and diabetes camps can be very important in helping teenagers cope with their diabetes, drawing strength from adult role models with diabetes who serve as staff and from each other.

• Reward good diabetes control with greater privileges. One of the most important privileges to a teenager is driving a car. Explain that driving, in particular, requires good control of diabetes. (Remember that your child should always wear and carry diabetes identification while driving.)

• Discuss the use of cigarettes, alcohol, and drugs with your child, or have a member of your health team do so.

While you may not approve of these behaviors, your child needs to know how they affect his or her diabetes control. If your child sees these discussions as lectures on moral conduct, or if you have difficulty bringing up the subject, arrange for the doctor or diabetes educator to have a more "objective" discussion with your child.

• Be realistic. Treating diabetes with insulin is not a perfect solution. Even intensive treatment programs, which are rarely possible to implement in children, cannot achieve perfectly normal control of the body's metabolism and blood sugar levels. If parents have unrealistic expectations, children may feel obligated to make up blood sugar test results to satisfy what they think is expected by their parents or doctors. Whatever you do, don't treat your child's diabetes diary as a report card. Rather, use it as a tool for interpreting his or her diabetes management.

The teen years are a time of growing independence. As a parent, you will need to gradually loosen the reins—even if it means sometimes standing by and watching as your child jeopardizes his or her diabetes control. On the other hand, don't make the mistake of dropping the reins altogether. Most teenagers are not yet capable of managing their diabetes all by themselves, even though they may give the impression that they are. Almost all instances of ketoacidosis in teenagers are a result of the child not taking one or more insulin injections.

A Family Affair

When a child has diabetes, everyone in the family will be touched in one way or another. It is perfectly normal to feel confused, sad, desperate, angry, guilty, and overwhelmed when your child is diagnosed with diabetes—if not right away, at some time after the diagnosis. Moreover, different adults may deal with their feelings in entirely different ways. For instance, a mother may cope by focusing all of her time and attention on keeping the diabetes under control, to the exclusion of others in the family, which could lead them to feel neglected. A father, thinking he must be strong, may hide his true feelings about the diagnosis, leading his partner to think that he's handling the diagnosis better than she is, or that he just doesn't care. You may feel that you should have been able to do something to prevent the diabetes, or that you are somehow responsible for it. (You should know that even if one side of the family *does* have diabetes, it appears that factors need to be inherited from *both* sides of the family to set the stage for the development of insulin-dependent diabetes.)

At the same time, you may be overwhelmed with information about diabetes and the various tasks necessary to manage the illness, such as blood glucose monitoring and giving insulin injections. You will also have to start making practical decisions about managing your child's diabetes: How will you divide up the day-to-day responsibilities of your child's diabetes care? How will you help your child cope with the diagnosis? How can you ensure that other children don't feel "left out"? And how will you handle the increased financial burden?

If you and your spouse or partner have already tackled serious problems together, you may be able to cope with this new situation on your own. It often takes professional counseling from a therapist, a certified diabetes educator, or another professional who is familiar with diabetes and its impact on the family. A therapist can help the entire family communicate their feelings and air their grievances in positive ways.

Even if you don't seek professional help, there are several ways to ease the strain of diabetes on your family:

• Share the responsibilities of diabetes care with your partner. Try not to let the burden of care fall on one person. If you are a single parent, you may be able to share the responsibility with the child's grandparents or an older brother or sister of the child. Divide up the daily responsibilities so that, for instance, one person gives or supervises the morning injection and the other handles the evening injection.

• Involve the other children. Letting other children help out—filling out the diabetes diary with blood sugar readings, or preparing a snack, for example—helps them feel more comfortable with their sibling's diabetes. It also helps the affected child feel more welcome and less of a burden on the family.

• Go to medical appointments together once or twice a year. When both of you talk with the doctor and ask questions, each parent or involved adult feels more informed and committed.

• Plan ways to cope with the increased expense. Explore programs of medical support for children with chronic health problems. You may qualify because of the cost of the problem even if you are not eligible for Medicaid.

Keeping family ties strong may be one of the best ways to help your child cope with diabetes. Studies have shown that children who have lots of family and professional support often have better control over their diabetes.

Above all, remember that a child with diabetes is, first of all, a child. He or she needs to be loved, disciplined, educated, and treated first as a child.

CHAPTER 12

Taking Charge of Your Diabetes

Now that you know how to live with diabetes, you need to know how to live *well*. Having a basic understanding of the disease, its potential complications and treatment is a good beginning. But it's just the beginning. Now you must learn to incorporate your new behaviors into your life for the rest of your days—and without letting your diabetes take control.

If you have recently been diagnosed, this may seem like a lofty goal. You're bound to feel overwhelmed with information and new tasks to perform, particularly if you (or a loved one) have insulin-dependent diabetes. The more quickly you master the basics—eating right, exercising regularly, monitoring blood sugar levels, injecting insulin, and so forth—the more quickly you will recognize that you are in control of this problem, and the more confidence you will have. Your health care team can be enormously helpful in these early weeks. Take advantage of their knowledge and expertise.

Remember, too, that it is impossible to learn in a few days or even weeks all you need to know about managing your diabetes and about coping with the many challenges it poses.

Initially, you will learn only those parts of diabetes care that are absolutely essential for managing your (or a loved one's) diabetes at home. Some skills you will learn only when a situation arises, since it is difficult to learn how to handle something you have never experienced.

It's perfectly normal to feel angry and resentful about your diagnosis, or simply deny it altogether. One of the first questions that may spring to mind is "Why me?" Or you may think it's not fair that you have to watch what you eat, control your weight, exercise, test your blood sugar, and possibly use medication to have what other people take for granted— good health. Keep in mind that, with the exception of monitoring your blood sugar and keeping records, you are not being asked to do much more than what *all* Americans are now encouraged to do to stay healthy. Even your motivation for making lifestyle changes is the same: avoiding such long-term problems as heart disease. The only difference is that you have a more immediate barometer of your health—your blood sugar levels.

Still, if you constantly feel as though you are being deprived of the good life, that the quality of your life has taken a decided turn for the worse now that you have diabetes, you should discuss your problems with your health care team, particularly if your feelings are interfering with your ability to take care of yourself. Your doctor or diabetes educator may be able to make some temporary allowances in your diabetes care plan to help you feel less deprived.

Members of your diabetes care team can also help you overcome or cope with some of your worst fears about diabetes: the long-term effects of diabetes on your health, how having diabetes will affect your work, whether or not you will be able to have children. (To make the best use of your diabetes care team, see "Getting the Most from Your Diabetes Care Team," on page 21.) Be sure to mention to your doctor or diabetes educator things you may have heard about diabetes from relatives, friends, or other sources. Much of what you have heard may not apply to you, may be out of date, or may simply be untrue! Keep in mind, too, that there is almost nothing a person with diabetes can't do that other children and adults do, *provided the diabetes is taken care of.*

A key to successful management of your diabetes is to be realistic about your diabetes and what you and your treatment team can accomplish. Remember, even the most intensive insulin regimens can't mimic the body's finely tuned system of adjusting insulin to meet ever-changing needs. So if you take diabetes medication and expect to record "perfect scores" on your glucose monitoring tests, you may be in for a disappointment. Nor should glucose test results be used as a "report card" of success or failure in the management of your diabetes. Rather, sustained high blood sugar levels or large swings in blood sugar levels are a sign that you and your treatment team need to adjust your treatment plan.

Remember, too, that as much as the treatment of diabetes has improved over the past ten years, there's no absolute guarantee that you *won't* develop complications later on— even if your diabetes is well controlled. On the other hand, as was pointed out in Chapter 8, we know that people with poorly controlled diabetes generally develop complications sooner than people whose diabetes is better controlled. So do your best to keep your diabetes under control. What we don't know is exactly why some people are able to achieve better control than others. The people who take very poor care of their diabetes and are more likely to get early complications probably won't be reading this or any other guidebook. But for the many who try their best, results may vary. So don't blame yourself if you develop complications. It's hard enough to deal with complications without the added guilt that you could have or *should* have prevented them.

If you slip up on your treatment plan now and then (which is bound to happen), don't throw up your hands and give up altogether. Instead, start anew the next day. You may also want to sit down with your doctor or diabetes educator and ask for some general guidelines about handling special situations, such as holidays, sleeping late, or occasionally having a drink or two at a party.

Your long-term objective is to live *with* diabetes, not *for* it. This means that you shouldn't deny or ignore your diabetes, nor should it become an obsession—or an excuse for not living your life to the fullest. You'll have to learn to strike a balance between taking care of your diabetes and keeping it always in the back of your mind, and not letting it interfere with what you want to accomplish in life.

Above all, remember: nothing you or a loved one did caused the diabetes, and nothing you can do will cure it. You can, however, do much to control your diabetes, feel better physically and emotionally, and improve the quality of your life—and this can be very empowering. In fact, because you have a strong motivation to take care of yourself, you are more likely to be in better health—and feel better about yourself—than many people who *don't* have diabetes.

Epilogue:
Hope for the Future

In 1922 a young British medical student suspected that his symptoms—frequent urination, excessive thirst, weight loss, and weakness—might be due to diabetes. He confirmed his suspicion with a urine test that revealed a large amount of sugar in his urine. To spare his family the agony of watching him waste away and die, he went to the the south of Italy to spend his last months. When he arrived, he found a telegram instructing him to rush back because insulin was available. He returned home for treatment and went on to live a long and productive life over the next 60 years as a world famous diabetes specialist and researcher. He'd benefitted from the first miracle in the battle to conquer diabetes—insulin. Since that time, many discoveries and developments have helped us to understand more about how diabetes develops and to better treat it. There is more research about diabetes going on today than ever before, so there is every reason to expect a brighter outlook for people with diabetes in the years to come.

As we mentioned in Chapter 2, researchers now recognize that insulin-dependent diabetes is an autoimmune disease in which the body's own immune defense system for some reason attacks and destroys the insulin-producing beta cells in the pancreas. This discovery has led to the testing of large numbers of relatives of people with diabetes and others, to find people who have the antibodies associated with the later development of diabetes. This kind of screening test, together with blood tests that demonstrate that the beta cells are losing their ability to produce enough insulin, has led to another avenue of research that holds promise of preventing insulin-dependent diabetes altogether. Researchers at the University of Florida and elsewhere are now attempting to prevent the development of diabetes in susceptible people by giving them medications that suppress the autoimmune process.

This research will not, of course, affect people who already have diabetes. It can, however, be important for the siblings or children of people with insulin-dependent diabetes, who have a two to five percent change of developing the disease.

Other promising developments for the treatment of people with diabetes include the following:

Insulin pills: Taking the insulin capsule or pill just before meals would certainly be easier than giving yourself an insulin injection. Insulin pills would actually work better than injected insulin, too, because the drug would be absorbed into the gastrointestinal tract and go first to the liver, as does the insulin secreted by the pancreas. Unfortunately, insulin in its present form is broken down in the digestive tract like any other protein, and digested. Research is now under way to find ways to protect insulin from destruction by the digestive tract so that it can be absorbed into the bloodstream. This would be a terrific breakthrough.

Artificial pancreas: Such a device would continuously measure blood glucose levels and send information to a pump that would inject either insulin or glucagon into the bloodstream to control blood sugar levels. The main problem with such a system is finding a way to continuously measure blood glucose. Placing a sensor directly into the bloodstream carries the risk of infection and blood clots, and placing a sensor anywhere else on the body causes scarring and does not provide accurate information. Researchers are currently looking into a laser method for measuring blood glucose that would not require contact with blood or tissue fluids.

Transplants: Numerous animal and human transplants of either the entire pancreas, a part of the pancreas, or the insulin-producing beta cells, have been successfully carried out. The problem with transplantation is that it requires taking powerful immunosuppressive drugs for the rest of your life so that the transplant will not be rejected. This makes sense if a person is having a kidney transplant because the benefits of the transplant outweigh the risks of the immunosuppressive drugs. Transplantation does not yet make sense for most people with diabetes, who can safely and effectively control their diabetes with diet, exercise, and insulin. There is also the problem of obtaining enough donor pancreases or beta cells to perform transplantations of many people with diabetes. (There are probably half a million people with insulin-dependent diabetes in the United States alone.)

Researchers are now experimenting with the possibility of transplanting animal beta cells encased in membranes that protect them from immune rejection but that permit glucose and insulin to pass through. Other scientists are investigating the feasibility of growing beta cells in the laboratory in large numbers for transplantation.

Finally, scientists are looking further into the causes and prevention of complications. We now recognize that high blood sugar levels cause changes in connective tissue and other proteins in the body, resulting in long-term complications. How can high blood sugar cause complications when the sugar is in the blood and can't get into the tissues without the help of insulin? These complications occur in tissues that do not depend on insulin for glucose absorption—the kidney, the nervous system, the retina of the eye, and the blood vessel walls—yet receive as much sugar as is in the bloodstream.

So why doesn't everyone who has an elevated blood sugar level develop complications? Research is now under way to determine how various people handle the changes in connective tissue that result from high blood sugar levels. Once these differences are understood, it may be possible to administer chemicals that interrupt the accumulation of damaging substances in suspectible people.

As you can see, the future holds much promise for people with diabetes. In the meantime, try to do the best you can managing your diabetes so you can take advantage of these new developments in the years to come.

Recommended Resources

The more you know about diabetes, the more you will want to know. The following organizations can provide you with more information and support.

Diabetes Care and Support

American Diabetes Association
National Service Center
1660 Duke Street
Alexandria, VA 22314
(800) 232-3472

This voluntary health organization is dedicated to increasing public awareness of diabetes and promoting and supporting diabetes research. The ADA publishes exchange lists for meal planning, along with numerous other pamphlets, booklets, and books, most available for a nominal fee. The organization also compiles an annual *Buyer's Guide to Diabetes*

Products, which reviews a wide range of diabetes products and insulin. For a modest annual membership fee ($24 at this writing), you'll receive *Diabetes Forecast*, a monthly magazine full of helpful information and tips for people with diabetes and their families. Your membership also entitles yOu to discounts on all other ADA publications, access to the ADA's toll-free information hotline, and a host of other member benefits. In addition, the ADA supports diabetes camps around the country for children with diabetes, and provides referrals to physicians and other health care professionals who specialize in the treatment of people with diabetes. Look in the phone book for a local affiliate, or write or call the national office for more information and a publication list.

National Diabetes Information Clearinghouse
Box NDIC, 9000 Rockville Pike
Bethesda, MD 20892
(301) 468-2162

This publicly funded clearinghouse, part of the National Institute of Diabetes and Digestive and Kidney Diseases, was established to increase knowledge about diabetes among patients, health professionals, and the public. The organization provides pamphlets and booklets on diabetes care for patients and their families free or for a nominal fee. The clearinghouse maintains a current list of cookbooks for people with diabetes, as well as lists of publications on foot care, pregnancy, and kidney disease. Publications available free of charge include "Dental Tips for Diabetics" (also available in Spanish), "Diabetic Retinopathy," "Diet and Exercise in Noninsulin-Dependent Diabetes," "Diabetes in Black Americans," and "Diabetes in Hispanics" (also available in Spanish), Write or call with your queries or for a complete publication list.

Juvenile Diabetes Foundation International
432 Park Avenue South
New York, NY 10016
(212) 889-7575

This private, voluntary organization provides information on insulin-dependent diabetes. Check the phone book for a local affiliate, or contact the national office in New York.

Diabetes Forum
c/o CompuServe
5000 Arlington Centre Boulevard
P.O. Box 20212
Columbus, OH 43220
(614) 457-8650

If you have a computer with a modem and subscribe to the information data base CompuServe, you can join the Diabetes Forum. This is a network of people who have diabetes or an abiding interest in diabetes care and who communicate with each other via computer. Through the Diabetes Forum, you'll have access to a wealth of information and tips on diabetes care, as well as plenty of hand-holding from other members. Members can correspond directly through the Forum, asking questions, sharing their own experiences, and receiving invaluable support. The Forum is free when you subscribe to CompuServe (look in the computer section of your local bookstore or contact CompuServe at the above address), which charges a modest setup fee ($35 at this writing) and a monthly user's fee (about $2 per month).

Nutrition and Weight Control

American Dietetic Association
National Center for Nutrition and Dietetics

216 West Jackson Boulevard, Suite 800
Chicago, IL 60606-6995
(312) 899-0040

This professional organization can help you locate a qualified dietitian or nutrition counselor in your area.

Weight Watchers International
Jericho Atrium
500 North Broadway
Jericho, NY 11753-2196
(516) 939-0400

This organization hosts group meetings that offer a nutritionally sound weight-loss program as well as plenty of emotional support. Look in the phone book for a local affiliate or
contact Weight Watchers International for more information.

Taking Off Pounds Sensibly (TOPS) Club
4575 South Fifth St.
P.O. Box 07360
Milwaukee, WI 53207
(414) 482-4620

This organization provides group therapy for people who
want to lose weight. Members are required to use physician-
approved individual eating plans and physician-set weight-
loss goals. Check your phone directory for a local chapter or
write to the national office at the above address.

Overeaters Anonymous
P.O. Box 92870
Los Angeles, CA 90009

This support group for compulsive overeaters is based on
the twelve-step program of Alcoholics Anonymous. Check
the phone book for local groups.

Other Organizations

National Eye Institute
Building 31, Room 6A32
National Institutes of Health
9000 Rockville Pike
Bethesda, MD 20892
(301) 496-5248

This branch of the National Institutes of Health provides information on diabetes and eye disease.

National Heart, Lung and Blood Institute
Building 31, Room 4A21
National Institutes of Health
9000 Rockville Pike
Bethesda, MD 20892
(301) 496-4236

This branch of the National Institutes of Health has a variety of books and pamphlets on the prevention of heart disease. Write or call for a publication list.

American Heart Association
National Center
7320 Greenville Avenue
Dallas, TX 75231
(800) 242-8721

The AHA has a wealth of materials on low-fat, low-sodium eating, and other ways to reduce your risk of heart disease. Contact the national center or look in the phone book for the number of a local affiliate.

Medic Alert
Medic Alert Foundation International

Turlock, CA 95381-1009
(800) ID-ALERT (432-5378)

This nonprofit foundation manufactures jewelry and wallet cards that alert medical personnel and others to your medical condition. The organization also operates a twenty-four-hour hotline that provides medical professionals around the world with access to computerized medical information about you.

Recommended Reading

Cookbooks

American Diabetes Association/American Dietetic Association Family Cookbook, Volumes I, II, and III, by the American Diabetes Association and the American Dietetic Association (Prentice-Hall, 1987). Each volume offers more than 200 kitchen-tested recipes that the whole family will enjoy, as well as nutrition information and tips on eating out, losing weight, and saving time and money in the kitchen. These cookbooks may be ordered through the American Diabetes Association (address on page 187).

American Diabetes Association Holiday Cookbook, by Betty Wedman, M.S., R.D. (American Diabetes Association, 1986). Includes recipes for traditional Thanksgiving, Christmas, and Hanukkah celebrations and other special occasions. This cookbook may be ordered through the American Diabetes Association (address on page 187).

Cookbooks for People with Diabetes: Selected Annotations, prepared by the National Diabetes Information Clearinghouse. U.S. Department of Health and Human Services, Public Health Service, National Institute of Diabetes and Digestive and Kidney Diseases (NIH Publication No. 88-2177, 1988). This helpful bibliography lists close to 100 cookbooks for people with diabetes, many of which you won't find in the bookstore. The bibliography provides information about the price, source, and availability of each item. To order the bibliography, contact the National Diabetes Information Clearinghouse (address on page 188).

For Children with Diabetes and Their Families

Children with Diabetes (American Diabetes Association, 1986). Essential for parents, teachers, and others who work with children with diabetes. The book covers day-to-day diabetes management, as well as tips for meeting children's psychological needs. This book may be ordered through the American Diabetes Association.

Glossary

Acesulfame: An alternative sweetener (marketed as Sweet One or Sunett) that passes through the body without being metabolized and doesn't affect blood sugar levels. Unlike aspartame, it isn't affected by cooking.

Aspartame: An alternative sweetener (better known by the brand name NutraSweet) consisting of two amino acids that are digested as proteins and hence don't affect blood sugar levels. The sweetener is widely used in prepared foods and beverages, but because it is unstable at high temperatures and loses its sweet flavor, tabletop forms of aspartame cannot be used in cooking.

Beta islet cells: The insulin-producing cells in the pancreas.

Blood glucose tests: Blood tests used to measure blood sugar levels and to screen for and diagnose diabetes. The tests may be administered either before or after eating *(random* *blood glucose test)* or after an overnight fast *(fasting blood glucose test)*. See also *oral glucose tolerance test.*

Cholesterol: A fatty substance found in all animal fats and in every cell in the human body. Cholesterol plays a key role in the formation of cell membranes and in the manufacture of certain hormones. High blood levels of a type of cholesterol known as low-density lipoprotein (LDL) cholesterol are associated with an increased risk of heart disease.

Coronary heart disease: Progressive narrowing of the blood vessels that nourish the heart muscle, caused by a buildup of fat deposits, calcium, fibrous material, and other substances.

Diabetes mellitus: A chronic medical condition characterized by abnormally high blood sugar (glucose) levels resulting either from a lack of the hormone *insulin* or from an inability of the body to use insulin efficiently. There are two major forms of diabetes. Type I, or insulin-dependent diabetes, typically develops before age thirty. People with this disorder produce little or no insulin and must take insulin injections to control blood sugar levels. Type II, or non-insulin-dependent diabetes, usually develops in adulthood (after age forty). In many people with non-insulin-dependent diabetes, the pancreas produces insulin, but the body somehow becomes resistant to insulin's ability to help tissues absorb glucose from the bloodstream. The single most important risk factor for non-insulin-dependent diabetes is obesity, affecting some 80 percent of those with this type of diabetes, and the disease can often be controlled through weight-loss measures.

Diabetic coma: See *diabetic ketoacidosis* and *hypersomolar coma.*

Diabetic ketoacidosis: A life-threatening condition associated with uncontrolled insulin-dependent diabetes in which glucose and ketones, breakdown products of fats, build up in the bloodstream. Symptoms include a fruity breath odor, nausea and vomiting, shortness of breath, mental confusion, and, if left untreated, coma. Treatment includes the administration of insulin and fluids and, if necessary, hospitalization to treat the resulting dehydration and mineral imbalances.

Diabetic macular edema: A thickening of the *macula*, the small yellow spot on the retina (the part of the eye containing millions of light-sensitive cells that are essential for vision). The macula is the part of the retina where vision is sharpest.

Diabetic retinopathy: A type of eye disease affecting the small blood vessels in the eye among people with diabetes. The condition is characterized by a weakening and ballooning of the walls of the tiny blood vessels in the eye. Some blood vessels may become blocked altogether, cutting off the blood supply to the retina, the part of the eye containing millions of light-sensitive cells that are essential for vision. If retinopathy progresses to the *proliferative* stage, new blood vessels and fibrous tissue form on the retina, causing bleeding. If bleeding is severe, a sudden and painless loss of vision occurs.

Diabetologist: A physician who specializes in the treatment and care of people with diabetes.

Exchange system: A form of meal planning developed by the American Diabetes Association, the American Dietetic Association, and the U.S. Public Health Service to help people with diabetes and others interested in good nutrition eat healthfully. The program features a number of *exchange lists*, each comprised of foods containing approximately the same number of calories, carbohydrate, protein, fat, vitamins, minerals, and fiber. There are six exchange lists: the bread/starch exchange list, the meat exchange list, the vegetable exchange list, the fruit exchange list, the milk exchange list, and the fat exchange list.

Fasting blood glucose test: See *blood glucose tests*.

Fructose: A simple sugar that contains the same amount of calories as sucrose (table sugar), but is sweeter and is absorbed more slowly by the gastrointestinal tract. Fructose is one of many alternative sweeteners available to people with diabetes.

Gestational diabetes: A form of diabetes that occurs only during pregnancy (usually after the twenty-eighth week of pregnancy) and disappears after the baby is born. Women who develop gestational diabetes are at a greater risk of developing overt diabetes within five to ten years.

Gingivitis: An early and reversible form of gum disease in which the soft tissues surrounding the teeth become inflamed. Symptoms include bleeding gums on brushing the teeth, a bad taste in the mouth, and pain when chewing.

Glucagon: A hormone secreted by the alpha islet cells of the pancreas that releases stored sugars from the liver and other tissues into the bloodstream, helping to raise blood sugar levels. A form of injectable glucagon is used in the treatment of severe hypoglycemia.

Glucose: A form of sugar that circulates in the bloodstream. Glucose is a major source of energy for the body.

Glucose tolerance test: See *oral glucose tolerance test*.

Glycosylated hemoglobin test: A blood test used to measure the amount of sugar that has attached to the hemoglobin portion of the body's red blood cells over the previous one- to two-month period. The test, also known as the *hemoglobin A-1C test,* is used as a measure of long-term blood sugar control.

Honeymoon phase: A stage of insulin-dependent diabetes that occurs after treatment has begun in which the pancreas temporarily starts producing insulin again. The honeymoon phase may last anywhere from a few weeks to many months, and may be prolonged by taking enough insulin to maintain very good diabetes control.

Hyperglycemia: Abnormally high blood sugar levels (usually above 240 mg/dl) associated with poorly controlled diabetes.

Hypersomolar coma: Also known as hypersomolar hypoketotic coma. This condition occurs in people with non-insulin dependent diabetes when very high blood glucose levels combine with dehydration due to inadequate fluid intake, resulting in decreased circulation to the brain and coma.

Hypertension: Excessive force of blood in the arteries as it is pumped through the body. If left untreated, high blood pressure can increase the risk of eye disease, kidney problems, coronary heart disease, and stroke. Treatment measures include following a low-salt diet, losing weight, and, if necessary, taking antihypertension medications.

Hypoglycemia: Abnormally low blood sugar levels (usually below 70 mg/dl in people with diabetes) associated with the use of insulin or oral hypoglycemic medications. Symptoms include excessive hunger, sweating, shakiness, heart palpitations, disorientation, and confusion. If left untreated, the condition may cause loss of consciousness. Treatment involves consuming a sugar-containing food or beverage, such as hard candy, orange juice, or a regular (nondiet) soft drink. Severe episodes of hypoglycemia may require administration of a *glucagon* injection, which causes stored sugars in the liver to be released into the bloodstream.

Hypoglycemic unawareness: Decreased awareness of the symptoms of hypoglycemia (such as shakiness, sweating, and a racing heart) caused by absence of an adrenaline response (heart pounding, tightness in the chest, cold sweat, trembling).

Impaired glucose tolerance: Blood sugar levels that are higher than normal (115 mg/dl or more fasting and more than 140 mg/dl one and two hours after a glucose load [see *oral glucose tolerance test*]) but lower than those used to diagnose diabetes mellitus (140 mg/dl or more fasting and 200 mg/dl or more after a glucose load). About 25 percent of people with IGT eventually develop diabetes.

Insensitive feet: Loss of feeling in the feet, usually caused by a combination of circulatory problems and nerve damage in the feet of people with long-standing diabetes.

Insulin: A hormone secreted by beta islet cells of the pancreas gland, just behind the stomach. Insulin helps the body's tissues store and use the glucose, protein, and fats circulating in the bloodstream after a meal.

Insulin-dependent diabetes: See *diabetes mellitus.*

Insulin infuser: A device consisting of a plastic tube that is inserted into the fatty tissue just under the skin, through which insulin injections are administered.

Insulin pen: A device that looks like a cartridge pen but instead is equipped with a needle and insulin cartridges. Convenient for insulin users who are visually impaired or who take more than two insulin shots a day.

Insulin pump: Computerized device that delivers regulated, steady amounts of insulin into the bloodstream via a plastic tube and needle inserted under the fatty layer of skin. The device can be manipulated to deliver bursts of insulin for meals and snacks.

Insulin reaction: See *hypoglycemia*.

Insulin resistance: A condition in which the body does not use insulin efficiently, either because the insulin does not bind to the cell as a result of problems with insulin receptors on the surface of the cell, or because, once bound to the cell, insulin cannot exert its usual actions.

Insulin shock: See *hypoglycemia*.

Islets of Langerhans: Specialized cells in the pancreas that secrete various hormones associated with the regulation of glucose levels in the bloodstream, including *insulin* (from beta islet cells), which helps lower blood sugar levels, and *glucagon* (from alpha islet cells), which stimulates the release of sugars stored in the liver and raises blood sugar levels.

Jet injector: A device that delivers insulin into the body by using pressure to send a stream of insulin solution through the skin.

Ketones: Breakdown products of fats that form when the body needs to use fat for fuel. Without insulin, the body cannot use ketones for fuel, and the substances build up in the bloodstream, spilling over into the urine. If left untreated, the buildup of ketones in the bloodstream can lead to a life-threatening condition known as *diabetic ketoacidosis*.

Laser photocoagulation: A treatment in which a laser beam is used to burn spots on the retina, which prevents the progression of *diabetic retinopathy*.

Lipodystrophy: A loss or excess accumulation of fat tissue that sometimes forms at the site of insulin injections.

Non-insulin-dependent diabetes: See *diabetes mellitus*.

Ophthalmologist: A physician who specializes in the medical and surgical treatment of eye disease. (Note: an *optician* is a person who fits eyeglasses and contact lenses by prescription; an *optometrist* is a licensed specialist who can perform an eye examination and can prescribe corrective lenses but cannot treat diabetic eye disease.)

Oral glucose tolerance test: A type of blood glucose test used to determine how the body responds to an increase in blood sugar. Blood glucose is measured before the patient consumes a concentrated glucose drink, and again one and two hours later.

Oral hypoglycemic medications: Drugs in the form of pills that are given to people with non-insulin-dependent diabetes to help lower blood sugar levels. (Only *sulfonylureas* are available in the U.S. Another class of drugs, *phenformins*, is used elsewhere.)

Orthostatic hypotension: A drop in blood pressure on standing or sitting up that may cause dizziness and, in severe cases, fainting.

Pancreas: The gland just behind the stomach which makes enzymes and hormones responsible for helping the body digest and process food. The pancreas secretes pancreatic juice, which contains several digestive enzymes, directly into the small intestine (where food is digested). It also secretes the hormones *insulin* and *glucagon* from specialized *islets of Langerhans* cells directly into the bloodstream, where these hormones help regulate blood sugar levels.

Periodontal disease: Gum disease. (See also *gingivitis* and *periodontitis.)*

Periodontitis: An advanced form of gum disease in which the supporting ligaments and bony socket of the tooth become infected, often leading to tooth loss.

Podiatrist: A licensed specialist who is able to diagnose and treat (with prescription medication and surgery) foot problems.

Preeclampsia: High blood pressure, accompanied by protein in the urine and water retention, that sometimes develops during the latter half of pregnancy. Treatment involves bed rest, antihypertensive medication, and, if preeclampsia is severe, preterm delivery of the baby.

Random blood glucose test: See *blood glucose tests.*

Saccharin: A zero-calorie sweetener that doesn't affect blood sugar levels. The sweetener is stable at high temperatures and can be used in cooking, but often has a bitter aftertaste.

SMBG tests: Self-monitoring blood glucose tests that use chemically treated strips which react with glucose in blood. The strip changes color and can be compared to a standard color chart or read by a meter. The tests permit patients to estimate blood sugar levels at any time of the day.

Sucrose: Table sugar, made up of two linked sugar molecules.

Sulfonylureas: Oral medications given to people with non-insulin-dependent diabetes to help lower blood sugar levels. (One class of *oral hypoglycemic medications.*)

Triglycerides: A type of fat that circulates in the bloodstream and is either used as energy or stored in the body's tissues as fat. Triglycerides can be manufactured by the liver and also come from the fat in foods. High levels may increase the risk of heart disease.

Type I Diabetes: See *diabetes mellitus.*

Type II Diabetes: See *diabetes mellitus.*

Appendix

Suggested Weights for Adults (USDA, 1990)

Height[a]	Weight in Pounds[b]	
	19 to 34 years	*35 years and over*
5'0"	97–128[c]	108–138
5'1"	101–132	111–143
5'2"	104–137	115–148
5'3"	107–141	119–152
5'4"	111–146	122–157
5'5"	114–150	126–162
5'6"	118–155	130–167
5'7"	121–160	134–172
5'8"	125–164	138–178
5'9"	129–169	142–183
5'10"	132–174	146–188
5'11"	136–179	151–194
6'0"	140–184	155–199
6'1"	144–189	159–205
6'2"	148–195	164–210
6'3"	152–200	168–216
6'4"	156–205	173–222
6'5"	160–211	177–228
6'6"	164–216	182–234

[a]Without shoes.
[b]Without clothes.
[c]The higher weights in the ranges generally apply to men, who tend to have more muscle and bone; the lower weights more often apply to women, who have less muscle and bone.

Food Exchange Lists

The Exchange Lists are the basis of a meal planning system designed by a committee of the American Diabetes Association and the American Dietetic Association. While designed primarily for people with diabetes and others who must follow special diets, the Exchange Lists are based on principles of good nutrition that apply to everyone. Copyright © 1989 by American Diabetes Association, Inc., and the American Dietetic Association.

Bread/Starch Exchange

Each item in this list contains approximately 15 grams of carbohydrate, 3 grams of protein, a trace of fat, and 80 calories. Whole-grain products average about 2 grams of fiber per exchange. Some foods are higher in fiber. Those foods that contain 3 or more grams of fiber per exchange are identified with the fiber symbol ✲

You can choose your starch exchanges from any of the items on this list. If you want to eat a starch food that is not on this list, the general rule is that:

- ½ cup of cereal, grain, or pasta is one exchange.
- 1 ounce of a bread product is one exchange.

Your dietitian can help you be more exact.

CEREALS/GRAINS/PASTA

Bran cereals, concentrated (such as Bran Buds®, All-Bran®) ⋙	⅓ cup
Bran cereals, flaked ⋙	½ cup
Bulgur (cooked)	½ cup
Cooked cereals	½ cup
Cornmeal (dry)	2½ tbsp.
Grape-Nuts®	3 tbsp.
Grits (cooked)	½ cup
Other ready-to-eat unsweetened cereals	¾ cup
Pasta (cooked)	½ cup
Puffed cereal	1½ cup
Rice, white or brown (cooked)	⅓ cup
Shredded wheat	½ cup
Wheat germ ⋙	3 tbsp.

DRIED BEANS/PEAS/LENTILS

Beans and peas (cooked) (such as kidney, white, split, black-eyed) ⋙	⅓ cup
Lentils (cooked) ⋙	⅓ cup
Baked beans ⋙	¼ cup

STARCHY VEGETABLES

Corn ⋙	½ cup
Corn on cob, 6 in. long ⋙	1
Lima beans ⋙	½ cup
Peas, green (canned or frozen) ⋙	½ cup
Plantain ⋙	½ cup
Potato, baked	1 small (3 oz.)
Potato, mashed	½ cup
Squash, winter (acorn, butternut) ⋙	1 cup
Yam, sweet potato, plain	⅓ cup

⋙ *3 grams or more of fiber per exchange*

BREAD

Bagel	½ (1 oz.)
Bread sticks, crisp, 4 in. long × ½ in.	2 (⅔ oz.)
Croutons, low-fat	1 cup
English muffin	½
Frankfurter or hamburger bun	½ (1 oz.)
Pita, 6 in. across	½
Plain roll, small	1 (1 oz.)
Raisin, unfrosted	1 slice (1 oz.)
Rye, pumpernickel	1 slice (1 oz.)
Tortilla, 6 in. across	1
White (including French, Italian)	1 slice (1 oz.)
Whole wheat	1 slice (1 oz.)

CRACKERS/SNACKS

Animal crackers	8
Graham crackers, 2½ in. square	3
Matzoh	¾ oz.
Melba toast	5 slices
Oyster crackers	24
Popcorn (popped, no fat added)	3 cups
Pretzels	¾ oz.
Rye crisp, 2 in. × 3½ in. ✿	4
Saltine-type crackers	6
Whole-wheat crackers, no fat added (crisp breads, such as Finn®, Kavli®, Wasa®) ✿	2–4 slices (¾ oz.)

STARCH FOODS PREPARED WITH FAT
(count as 1 starch/bread exchange,
plus 1 fat exchange)

Biscuit, 2½ in. across	1
Chow mein noodles	½ cup
Corn bread, 2 in. cube	1 (2 oz.)
Cracker, round butter type	6
French-fried potatoes, 2 in. to 3½ in. long	10 (1½ oz.)
Muffin, plain, small	1
Pancake, 4 in. across	2

✿ *3 grams or more of fiber per exchange*

Stuffing, bread (prepared)	¼ cup
Taco shell, 6 in. across	2
Waffle, 4½ in. square	1
Whole-wheat crackers, fat added (such as Triscuit®) ᴥ	4–6 (1 oz.)

Meat Exchange

Each serving of meat and substitutes on this list contains about 7 grams of protein. The amount of fat and number of calories vary, depending on what kind of meat or substitute you choose. The list is divided into three parts based on the amount of fat and calories: lean meat, medium-fat meat, and high-fat meat. One ounce (one meat exchange) of each of these includes:

	Carbohydrate *(grams)*	Protein *(grams)*	Fat *(grams)*	Calories
Lean	0	7	3	55
Medium-fat	0	7	5	75
High-fat	0	7	8	100

You are encouraged to use more lean and medium-fat meat, poultry, and fish in your meal plan. This will help decrease your fat intake, which may help decrease your risk for heart disease. The items from the high-fat group are high in saturated fat, cholesterol, and calories. You should limit your choices from the high-fat group to three times per week. Meat and substitutes do not contribute any fiber to your meal plan.

ᴥ *3 grams or more of fiber per exchange*
◆ *Meats and meat substitutes that have 400 milligrams or more of sodium per exchange are indicated with this symbol.*
★ *Meats and meat substitutes that have 400 mg or more of sodium if two or more exchanges are eaten are indicated with this symbol.*

LEAN MEAT AND SUBSTITUTES
(One exchange is equal to any one of the following items)

Beef: USDA select or choice grades of lean beef, such as round, sirloin, and flank steak; tenderloin; and chipped beef ◆ — 1 oz.

Pork: Lean pork, such as fresh ham; canned, cured, or boiled ham ◆ ; Canadian bacon ◆ , tenderloin. — 1 oz.

Veal: All cuts are lean except for veal cutlets (ground or cubed). Examples of lean veal are chops and roasts. — 1 oz.

Poultry: Chicken, turkey, Cornish hen (without skin) — 1 oz.

Fish:
All fresh and frozen fish	1 oz.
Crab, lobster, scallops, shrimp, clams (fresh or canned in water)	2 oz.
Oysters	6 medium
Tuna ★ (canned in water)	¼ cup
Herring ★ (uncreamed or smoked)	1 oz.
Sardines (canned)	2 medium

Wild Game:
Venison, rabbit, squirrel	1 oz.
Pheasant, duck, goose (without skin)	1 oz.

Cheese:
Any cottage cheese ★	¼ cup
Grated parmesan	2 Tbsp.
Diet cheeses ◆ (with less than 55 calories per ounce)	1 oz.

Other:
95% fat-free luncheon meat ◆	1½ oz.
Egg whites	3 whites
Egg substitutes with less than 55 calories per ½ cup	½ cup

◆ *400 mg or more of sodium per exchange*
★ *400 mg or more of sodium if two or more exchanges are eaten*

MEDIUM-FAT MEAT AND SUBSTITUTES
(One exchange is equal to any one of the following items)

Beef: Most beef products fall into this category. 1 oz.
Examples are all ground beef, roast
(rib, chuck, rump), steak (cubed,
Porterhouse, T-bone), and meatloaf.

Pork: Most pork products fall into this 1 oz.
category. Examples are chops, loin
roast, Boston butt, cutlets.

Lamb: Most lamb products fall into this 1 oz.
category. Examples are chops, leg, and
roast.

Veal: Cutlet (ground or cubed, unbreaded) 1 oz.

Poultry: Chicken (with skin), domestic duck or 1 oz.
goose (well drained of fat), ground
turkey

Fish: Tuna ★ (canned in oil and drained) ¼ cup
Salmon ★ (canned) ¼ cup

Cheese: Skim or part-skim milk cheeses, such as:
Ricotta ¼ cup
Mozzarella 1 oz.
Diet cheeses ◆ (with 56–80 calories per 1 oz.
ounce)

Other: 86% fat-free luncheon meat ★ 1 oz.
Egg (high in cholesterol, limit to 3 per 1
week)
Egg substitutes with 56–80 calories per ¼ cup
¼ cup
Tofu (2½ in. × 2¾ in. × 1 in.) 4 oz.
Liver, heart, kidney, sweetbreads (high in 1 oz.
cholesterol)

◆ *400 mg or more of sodium per exchange*
★ *400 mg or more of sodium if two or more exchanges are eaten*

HIGH-FAT MEAT AND SUBSTITUTES

Remember, these items are high in saturated fat, cholesterol, and calories, and should be used only three times per week.

(One exchange is equal to any one of the following items)

Beef:	Most USDA prime cuts of beef, such as ribs, corned beef ★	1 oz.
Pork:	Spareribs, ground pork, pork sausage ◆ (patty or link)	1 oz.
Lamb:	Patties (ground lamb)	1 oz.
Fish:	Any fried fish product	1 oz.
Cheese:	All regular cheeses, such as American ◆, blue ◆, cheddar ★, Monterey jack ★, Swiss	1 oz.
Other:	Luncheon meat ◆, such as bologna, salami, pimiento loaf	1 oz.
	Sausage ◆, such as Polish, Italian smoked	1 oz.
	Knockwurst ◆	1 oz.
	Bratwurst ★	1 oz.
	Frankfurter ◆ (turkey or chicken)	1 frank (10/lb.)
	Peanut butter (contains unsaturated fat)	1 Tbsp.

Count as one high-fat meat plus one fat exchange:

	Frankfurter ◆ (beef, pork, or combination)	1 frank (10/lb.)

◆ *400 mg or more of sodium per exchange*
★ *400 mg or more of sodium if two or more exchanges are eaten*

Vegetable Exchange

Each vegetable serving on this list contains about 5 grams of carbohydrate, 2 grams of protein, and 25 calories. Vegetables contain 2 to 3 grams of dietary fiber. Vegetables which contain 400 mg or more of sodium per exchange are identified with a ◆ symbol.

Vegetables are a good source of vitamins and minerals. Fresh and frozen vegetables have more vitamins and less added salt. Rinsing canned vegetables will remove much of the salt.

Unless otherwise noted, the serving size for vegetables (one vegetable exchange) is:

½ cup of cooked vegetables or vegetable juice
1 cup of raw vegetables

Artichoke (½ medium)
Asparagus
Beans (green, wax, Italian)
Bean sprouts
Beets
Broccoli
Brussels sprouts
Cabbage, cooked
Carrots
Cauliflower
Eggplant
Greens (collard, mustard, turnip)
Kohlrabi
Leeks

Mushrooms, cooked
Okra
Onions
Pea pods
Peppers (green)
Rutabaga
Sauerkraut ◆
Spinach, cooked
Summer squash (crookneck)
Tomato (one large)
Tomato/vegetable juice ◆
Turnips
Water chestnuts
Zucchini, cooked

Starchy vegetables such as corn, peas, and potatoes are found on the Bread/Starch List.

For free vegetables, see Free Food List on page 215.

◆ *400 mg or more of sodium per exchange*

Fruit Exchange

Each item on this list contains about 15 grams of carbohydrate and 60 calories. Fresh, frozen, and dried fruits have about 2 grams of fiber per exchange. Fruits that have 3 or more grams of fiber per exchange have a ❧ symbol. Fruit juices contain very little dietary fiber.

The carbohydrate and calorie contents for a fruit exchange are based on the usual serving of the most commonly eaten fruits. Use fresh fruits or fruits frozen or canned without sugar added. Whole fruit is more filling than fruit juice and may be a better choice for those who are trying to lose weight. Unless otherwise noted, the serving size for one fruit exchange is:

> ½ cup of fresh fruit or fruit juice
> ¼ cup of dried fruit

FRESH, FROZEN, AND UNSWEETENED CANNED FRUIT

Apple (raw, 2 in. across)	1 apple
Applesauce (unsweetened)	½ cup
Apricots (medium, raw)	4 apricots
Apricots (canned)	½ cup, or 4 halves
Banana (9 in. long)	½ banana
Blackberries (raw) ❧	¾ cup
Blueberries (raw) ❧	¾ cup
Cantaloupe (5 in. across)	⅓ melon
(cubes)	1 cup
Cherries (large, raw)	12 cherries
Cherries (canned)	½ cup
Figs (raw, 2 in. across)	2 figs
Fruit cocktail (canned)	½ cup
Grapefruit (medium)	½ grapefruit
Grapefruit (segments)	¾ cup
Grapes (small)	15 grapes
Honeydew melon (medium)	⅛ melon
(cubes)	1 cup
Kiwi (large)	1 kiwi
Mandarin oranges	¾ cup

❧ *3 or more grams of fiber per exchange*

Mango (small)	½ mango
Nectarine (2½ in. across) ❧	1 nectarine
Orange (2½ in. across)	1 orange
Papaya	1 cup
Peach (2¾ in. across)	1 peach, or ¾ cup
Peaches (canned)	½ cup or 2 halves
Pear	½ large, or 1 small
Pears (canned)	½ cup, or 2 halves
Persimmon (medium, native)	2 persimmons
Pineapple (raw)	¾ cup
Pineapple (canned)	⅓ cup
Plum (raw, 2 in. across)	2 plums
Pomegranate ❧	½ pomegranate
Raspberries (raw) ❧	1 cup
Strawberries (raw, whole) ❧	1¼ cup
Tangerine (2½ in. across) ❧	2 tangerines
Watermelon (cubes)	1¼ cup

DRIED FRUIT

Apples ❧	4 rings
Apricots ❧	7 halves
Dates	2½ medium
Figs ❧	1½
Prunes ❧	3 medium
Raisins	2 Tbsp.

FRUIT JUICE

Apple juice/cider	½ cup
Cranberry juice cocktail	⅓ cup
Grapefruit juice	½ cup
Grape juice	⅓ cup
Orange juice	½ cup
Pineapple juice	½ cup
Prune juice	⅓ cup

❧ *3 or more grams of fiber per exchange*

Milk Exchange

Each serving of milk or milk products on this list contains about 12 grams of carbohydrate and 8 grams of protein. The amount of fat in milk is measured in percent of butterfat. The calories vary, depending on what kind of milk you choose. The list is divided into three parts based on the amount of fat and calories: skim/very-low-fat milk, low-fat milk, and whole milk. One serving (one milk exchange) of each of these includes:

	Carbohydrate (grams)	Protein (grams)	Fat (grams)	Calories
Skim/Very-low-fat	12	8	trace	90
Low-fat	12	8	5	120
Whole	12	8	8	150

Milk is the body's main source of calcium, the mineral needed for growth and repair of bones. Yogurt is also a good source of calcium. Yogurt and many dry or powdered milk products have different amounts of fat. If you have questions about a particular item, read the label to find out the fat and calorie content.

Milk is good to drink, but it can also be added to cereal and to other foods. Many tasty dishes such as sugar-free pudding are made with milk (see the Combination Foods list). Add life to plain yogurt by adding one of your fruit exchanges to it.

SKIM AND VERY-LOW-FAT MILK

skim milk	1 cup
½% milk	1 cup
1% milk	1 cup
low-fat buttermilk	1 cup
evaporated skim milk	½ cup
dry nonfat milk	⅓ cup
plain nonfat yogurt	8 oz.

LOW-FAT MILK

2% milk	1 cup fluid
plain low-fat yogurt (with added nonfat milk solids)	8 oz.

WHOLE MILK

The whole milk group has much more fat per serving than the skim and lowfat groups. Whole milk has more than 3¼% butterfat. Try to limit your choices from the whole milk group as much as possible.

whole milk	1 cup
evaporated whole milk	½ cup
whole plain yogurt	8 oz.

Fat Exchange

Each serving on the fat list contains about 5 grams of fat and 45 calories.

The foods on the fat list contain mostly fat, although some items may also contain a small amount of protein. All fats are high in calories and should be carefully measured. Everyone should modify fat intake by eating unsaturated fats instead of saturated fats. The sodium content of these foods varies widely. Check the label for sodium information.

UNSATURATED FATS

Avocado	⅛ medium
Margarine	1 tsp.
Margarine, diet ★	1 tbsp.
Mayonnaise	1 tsp.
Mayonnaise, reduced calorie ★	1 tbsp.
Nuts and Seeds:	
Almonds, dry roasted	6 whole
Cashews, dry roasted	1 tbsp.

◆ *400 mg or more of sodium per exchange*
★ *400 mg or more of sodium if two or more exchanges are eaten*

Pecans	2 whole
Peanuts	20 small or 10 large
Walnuts	2 whole
Other nuts	1 tbsp.
Seeds, pine nuts, sunflower (without shells)	1 tbsp.
Pumpkin seeds	2 tsp.
Oil (corn, cottonseed, safflower, soybean, sunflower, olive, peanut)	1 tsp.
Olives ★	10 small or 5 large
Salad dressing, mayonnaise-type	2 tsp.
Salad dressing, mayonnaise-type, reduced-calorie	1 tbsp.
Salad dressing (oil varieties) ★	1 tbsp.
Salad dressing, reduced-calorie ◆	2 tbsp.

(Two tablespoons of low-calorie salad dressing is a free food.)

SATURATED FATS

Butter	1 tsp.
Bacon ★	1 slice
Chitterlings	½ oz.
Coconut, shredded	2 tbsp.
Coffee whitener, liquid	2 tbsp.
Coffee whitener, powder	4 tsp.
Cream (light, coffee, table)	2 tbsp.
Cream, sour	2 tbsp.
Cream (heavy, whipping)	1 tbsp.
Cream cheese	1 tbsp.
Salt pork ★	¼ oz.

◆ *400 mg or more of sodium per exchange*
★ *400 mg or more of sodium if two or more exchanges are eaten*

FREE FOODS

A free food is any food or drink that contains less than 20 calories per serving. You can eat as much as you want of those items that have no serving size specified. You may eat two or three servings per day of those itmes that have a specific serving size. Be sure to spread them out through the day.

Drinks:
Bouillon ◆ or broth without fat
Bouillon, low-sodium
Carbonated drinks, sugar-free
Carbonated water
Club soda
Cocoa powder, unsweetened (1 tbsp.)
Coffee/Tea
Drink mixes, sugar-free
Tonic water, sugar-free

Nonstick pan spray

Fruit:
Cranberries, unsweetened (1/2 cup)
Rhubarb, unsweetened (1/2 cup)

Vegetables:
(raw, 1 cup)
Cabbage
Celery
Chinese cabbage ⁍
Cucumber
Green onion
Hot peppers
Mushrooms
Radishes
Zucchini ⁍

Salad greens:
Endive
Escarole
Lettuce
Romaine
Spinach

Sweet Substitutes:
Candy, hard, sugar-free
Gelatin, sugar-free
Gum, sugar-free
Jam/Jelly, sugar-free (less than 20 cal./2 tsp.)
Pancake syrup, sugar-free (1–2 tbsp.)
Sugar substitutes (saccharin, aspartame)
Whipped topping (2 tbsp.)

Condiments:
Catsup (1 tbsp.)
Horseradish
Mustard
Pickles ◆, dill, unsweetened
Salad dressing, low-calorie (2 tbsp.)
Taco sauce (3 tbsp.)
Vinegar

⁍ *3 grams or more of fiber per exchange*
◆ *400 mg or more of sodium per exchange*

Seasonings can be very helpful in making food taste better. Be careful of how much sodium you use. Read the label, and choose those seasonings that do not contain sodium or salt.

Basil (fresh)
Celery seeds
Chili powder
Chives
Cinnamon
Curry
Dill
Flavoring extracts (vanilla,
    almond, walnut, peppermint,
    butter, lemon, etc.)
Garlic
Garlic powder
Herbs
Hot pepper sauce
Lemon

Lemon juice
Lemon pepper
Lime
Lime juice
Mint
Onion powder
Oregano
Paprika
Pepper
Pimiento
Spices
Soy sauce ◆
Soy sauce ◆ , low-sodium ("lite")
Wine, used in cooking (1/4 cup)
Worcestershire sauce

◆ *400 mg or more of sodium per exchange*

COMBINATION FOODS

Much of the food we eat is mixed together in various combinations. These combination foods do not fit into only one exchange list. It can be quite hard to tell what is in a certain casserole dish or baked food item. This is a list of average values for some typical combination foods. This list will help you fit these foods into your meal plan. Ask your dietitian for information about any other foods you'd like to eat. The *American Diabetes Association/American Dietetic Association Family Cookbooks* and the *American Diabetes Association Holiday Cookbook* have many recipes and further information about many foods, including combination foods. Check your library or bookstore.

Food	Amount	Exchanges
Casseroles, homemade	1 cup (8 oz.)	2 starch, 2 medium-fat meat, 1 fat
Cheese pizza ◆, thin crust	¼ of 15 oz. or ¼ of 10 in.	2 starch, 1 medium-fat meat, 1 fat
Chili with beans ☚, ◆ (commercial)	1 cup (8 oz.)	2 starch, 2 medium-fat meat, 2 fat
Chow mein ◆ (without noodles or rice)	2 cups (16 oz.)	1 starch, 2 vegetable, 2 lean meat
Macaroni and cheese ◆	1 cup (8 oz.)	2 starch, 1 medium-fat meat, 2 fat
Soup:		
Bean ☚, ◆	1 cup (8 oz.)	1 starch, 1 vegetable, 1 lean meat
Chunky, all varieties ◆	10-¾ oz. can	1 starch, 1 vegetable, 1 medium-fat meat
Cream ◆ (made with water)	1 cup (8 oz.)	1 starch, 1 fat
Vegetable ◆ or broth-type ◆	1 cup (8 oz.)	1 starch

☚ *3 grams or more of fiber per exchange*
◆ *400 mg or more of sodium per exchange*

| Spaghetti and meatballs ◆ (canned) | 1 cup (8 oz.) | 2 starch, 1 medium-fat meat, 1 fat |
| Sugar-free pudding (made with skim milk) | ½ cup | 1 starch |

If beans are used as a meat substitute:

| Dried beans ⋗, peas ⋗, lentils ⋗ | 1 cup (cooked) | 2 starch, 1 lean meat |

FOODS FOR OCCASIONAL USE

Moderate amounts of some foods can be used in your meal plan, in spite of their sugar or fat content, as long as you can maintain blood glucose control. The following list includes average exchange values for some of these foods. Because they are concentrated sources of carbohydrate, you will notice that the portion sizes are very small. Check with your dietitian for advice on how often and when you can eat them.

Food	Amount	Exchanges
Angel food cake	½₁₂ cake	2 starch
Cake, no icing	½₁₂ cake, or a 3 in. square	2 starch, 2 fat
Cookies	2 small (1¾ in. across)	1 starch, 1 fat
Frozen fruit yogurt	⅓ cup	1 starch
Gingersnaps	3	1 starch
Granola	¼ cup	1 starch, 1 fat
Granola bars	1 small	1 starch, 1 fat
Ice cream, any flavor	½ cup	1 starch, 2 fat
Ice milk, any flavor	½ cup	1 starch, 1 fat
Sherbet, any flavor	¼ cup	1 starch
Snack chips ★, all varieties	1 oz.	1 starch, 2 fat
Vanilla wafers	6 small	1 starch

⋗ 3 grams or more of fiber per exchange
◆ 400 mg or more of sodium per exchange
★ 400 mg or more of sodium if two or more exchanges are eaten

Diabetes Diary

Day/ Date	Insulin or Pills				Blood Glucose Tests		Urine Ketone Tests		Notes
	Time/Type/Dose				Time/Results		Time/Results		

Index

Stretching exercise, 62
Stroke, 40, 56, 116
  early warning signs, 119–20
Sugar
  in diet, 23
  processing, by body, 8–10
  refined vs. simple, 27
  table, 31, 106, 109, 203
  See also Blood glucose levels; Glucose
Sugar substitutes, 31–32
  and pregnancy, 149
Sulfa drug allergies, 68
Sulfonylureas, 67, 69–70, 202, 203
  See also Oral hypoglycemic agents
Support groups, 21
Surgery, 9, 74, 159–62
Sweating, 63, 70, 103–04, 109, 122
Sweets, 3, 5, 31–32
Swimming, 59–60, 64
Syringes, 79–81
  alternatives to, 79
  disposing of, 90–91, 165
  getting right size, 79
  and insulin concentrations, 78
  and travel, 163–66
Systolic pressure, 119

Target heart range, 61
Team sports, 59–60
Teen support groups, 175
Teeth and gums, 137–40
Tegretol, 121
Tests
  blood glucose, 92–99, 195–96
  by doctor, 92–93
  at home, 94–99
  kidney, 125–26
  prenatal, 149–51
  and travel, 165
  See also Monitoring; specific tests
Tetracycline, 123
Therapist, 21
Thiazides, 16, 73
Thirst, 10, 11, 14, 110, 112, 168
Thyroid problems, 70
Tolazamide, 69
Tolbutamide, 69
Tolinase, 69
TOPS (Taking Off Pounds Sensibly) Club, 48
Travel, 162–65
  and insulin concentrations, 78
  and monitoring, 105–06
  supplies, 165–67
Triglycerides, 8, 75, 117–18, 204
  and alcohol, 43
  and medication, 72
Turkey, 34
Type I diabetes. *See* Insulin-dependent diabetes
Type II diabetes. *See* Non-insulin-dependent diabetes

U-40 insulin bottles, 78
U-40 syringes, 78
U-100 insulin bottles, 78, 86
  and travel, 164
U-100 syringes, 78, 86

Ultralente (U), 76
Ultrasound, 150
Unconsciousness, 107, 110
U. S. Dietary Guidelines for Americans, 23, 40
U. S. Food and Drug Administration, 38
U. S. Public Health Service, 45
Unstable diabetes, 12–13
Upper-body exercises, 60
Ureters, 125
Uric acid concentrations, 49, 69
Urinalysis, 125
Urinary tract infections, 17, 123, 126–27
Urination, frequent, 1, 10, 11, 14, 110, 112, 168
Urine tests, 94, 97–99
  glucose, 94, 98
  ketone, 98, 111, 147, 154
  protein, 143

Vaginal lubrication problems, 124
Vascular surgeon, 133
Vegans, 36–37
Vegetable oils, 34
Vegetables, 27–28, 40, 42, 53
  exchange list, 46, 213
  high-fiber, 30, 51
  proteins, 37
  sauces for, 36
Vegetarians, 36–39
Viruses, 12
Vision problems, 11, 14, 110, 112, 130, 168
  testing, 94–95
  See also Eyes
Vitamin and mineral supplements, 37, 41, 48–49
Vitamin B-6, 122
Vitamin B$_{12}$, 37
Vitamin C, 37, 98
Vitamins, 28, 29, 34, 35, 40–41
Vomiting, 70, 110, 112–13, 123, 168

Walking, 59–60, 64–65, 149
Warm-up exercise, 62
Water, 41–42, 63
Water-insoluble fiber, 28–29
Water-soluble fiber, 28–29
Weakness, 109, 112, 168
Weight control, 16, 74, 126
  and alcohol, 43
  diet for, 24, 26, 46–51
  and exercise, 56
  and vitamin supplements, 41
Weight lifting, 60, 130
Weight loss, as symptom, 1, 10, 14
Weight Watchers, 21, 48, 190
Whole-grains, 27, 28, 37, 48
Women, 84. *See also* Pregnancy
Wounds, slow-healing, 14, 110
Wygesic, 121

X-ray dyes, 127

Yeast infection, 14
Yoga, 60, 130, 169

Zinc, 83
Zocor, 118